MW01034761

Kidney Stones Explained

DK Guyer, PhD

Copyright © 2020 – DK Guyer, PhD

All rights reserved. No part of this book may be used or reproduced in any manner, stored in a retrieval system, or transmitted in any form or by any means electronic, mechanical, photocopy, recording, scanning or any other except in the case of brief quotations in printed reviews, without prior written permission from the author or photocopied for personal use.

The contents of this book reflect the author's opinions, thoughts, observations, and conclusions, and serve only as informational and educational material. It is not intended as medical advice, medical diagnosis, or medical treatment. Everyone involved in the publishing is aware that its contents are only for informational and educational purposes. The author is not prescribing medical treatment nor attempting to negate current medical treatment. Should readers choose to follow any of the author's recommendations, without the supervision of a medical doctor, they are doing so at their own risk. Should readers decide to implement any of the information in this book, they are solely responsible for any outcome.

ISBN– 978-1-7332202-17

Printed in the United States of America

Disclaimer from the Author

These statements have not been evaluated by the Food and Drug Administration. The products mentioned in this book are not intended to diagnose, treat, cure, or prevent any disease.

Only a licensed medical doctor can prescribe medical treatment. I am not a medical doctor and do not practice as a doctor; therefore, the contents of this book must be disclosed to you as only my opinions, my thoughts, my observations, and my conclusions. The information serves only as informational and educational material. It is not intended as medical advice, medical diagnosis, or medical treatment.

All people involved in the publishing and distribution of this book are aware that its contents are only for information and educational purposes. I am not prescribing medical treatment, nor am I attempting to negate your current medical treatment plan. Should you choose to follow any of my recommendations without the supervision of a medical doctor, you are doing so at your own risk.

Natural health protocol is information and education that is highly regarded in the majority of the world. In the United States, the idea of limiting one's toxic intake of manmade foodstuffs and achieving better health through vital nutrition is disregarded as a mainstream preventative approach to better health. Rather, health conditions are addressed by treating symptoms after issues occur.

Should you decide to implement any of the information in this book, you do so at your own risk and are solely responsible for any outcome.

*It is health that is real wealth
and not pieces of gold and silver.*

Mahatma Gandhi

Preface

After spending years educating people on the importance of nutrition, I have had the fortunate opportunity of hearing people speak candidly about a variety of health issues. Kidney stones and kidney health are a predominant subject with minimal real and truthful information available for addressing the cause of the problem and how to eliminate it.

The misunderstood and highly promoted idea that kidney stones are inherited from your parents is a rare occurrence, as you will learn in this book. Hearing that people lose their jobs because they are unable to work while enduring the excruciating pain of passing a kidney stone is deplorable.

Most astonishing, is the lack of knowledge that kidney stones are a physical announcement that more serious disease is on the horizon if eating habits and lifestyle remain the same. Developing kidney stones can significantly disrupt daily life.

The United States is internationally recognized as the sickest, most undernourished and overfed nation in the world. Conflicting and often times inaccurate health education diminishes our ability to honor our bodies as the most valuable asset we will ever own.

In an age of convenient, synthetically altered food choices, statistics on disease and health conditions are growing at alarming rates. The medical community in the United States relies on prescription medications to the treat symptoms of health conditions. It has become my obligation to present truthful information to address and remove the cause of health concerns to gain and maintain better health.

Taking control of your health can reward you with many years of pain free days. I wish you the very best!

Table of Contents

CHAPTER 1

WHAT IS A KIDNEY STONE

Deposits of uric acid, minerals (such as calcium, magnesium, phosphorus, salts), and other toxins extracted from the blood collect inside the kidneys. Over time, stone-like composites can form when these minerals crystallize together.

Kidney stones are more prevalent in men than in women, with men developing them at an average rate of 19% in their lifetime. Women experience less than that with a 10% lifetime occurrence rate.[1]

The most interesting fact about kidney stones is understanding the underlying process that caused it to form.

We know that it occurs when a crystalline sediment remains unflushed from the kidney and accumulates, bonds together with other crystal and mineral elements to form one or more stones in one kidney rather than both.

It is my belief from years of observation that stones occur in only one kidney at a time because if forms on the side you are most likely to sleep on! When discussing kidney stones, I often ask people if they spend more time at night sleeping on the same side as the kidney stone formed. The answer is nearly always a resounding, "Yes!"

Persons sleeping all night on their stomach or back do not experience the problem of kidney stones as often as side sleepers.

The pressure from the weight of the sleeping body restricts blood flow to the kidney for six to eight hours or longer each day. After experiencing one kidney stone, a reoccurrence in the same kidney can surface again.

CHAPTER 2

DIFFERENT TYPES OF STONES

There are four common types of kidney stones identified through analysis.

Uric Acid Stones: This type of stone develops slowly. It is often associated with consuming a diet high in meat and poultry, eating processed and fast foods while consuming low amounts of water. Uric acid stones can occur in both sexes but are more common in men.

Struvite Stones: These stones can form quickly as a result of a bacterial infection in the urinary tract. Intense infections can create stones large enough to block kidney function and urine elimination. This type of stone is more prevalent among women. Struvite stones can be very dangerous.

Calcium Stones: These are much more common, but they tend to be a complicated mess! They can be made of composites containing calcium and oxalate crystals or calcium and phosphate amalgams or a combination of both types of calcium mixtures. To further muddle their complexity, nearly all of them begin as uric acid stones.

Calcium stones result from the consumption of high salt, high animal protein diets including bone broth powders and soups, high concentration of soybean and soybean oil products, high quantities of conventional dairy products, soda and energy drinks, and some prescription medications.

Cystine stones: These stones occur when the kidneys excrete elevated amounts of certain amino acids called cystine. They are less common and associated with cystinuria, a hereditary disorder.

CHAPTER 3

REDUCING THE RISK OF STONES

We know what causes kidney stones. Why are we still suffering from them? The answer is easy. It is easier to treat the resulting stone than to address the underlying cause.

Because no two persons consume the same amount of food, beverage, medication, or breathe the same toxins, kidney stones differ in their composition from person to person.

The scary part of this equation is that stones are a clear indication that the kidneys are compromised and struggling to do their job. Stones represent a symptom announcing that more extensive kidney disease is imminent unless food choices and lifestyle habits are altered. While it is a common belief that some people are predisposed to forming kidney stones, it is not an accurate statement unless they suffer a rare condition called cystinuria or are prone to certain urinary infections. Stones are formed as a direct result of what a person eats and drinks. The diet essentially expresses itself through painful stones.

**The kidneys process and filter approximately
50 gallons of blood a day.**

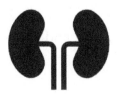

ACIDOSIS

The kidneys filter and remove waste from the blood. Without proper kidney function, all of the systems in the body become compromised and struggle to operate normally.

To illustrate the kidney's life-saving function, let's analyze what happens inside the body after consuming a slice of pepperoni pizza and soda. While it might have seemed like just a tasty lunch, it is an extraordinary toxic workload to the body. These products are unnatural and contain artificial preservatives, flavorings, colorings, synthetic ingredients, and are also high in fat, cholesterol, sugar, and create dehydration. As the pizza and soda make their way through the digestive system, several actions occur at once.

The liver metabolizes food components into usable nutrients, such as amino acid chains, vitamins, and minerals or waste. The metabolized elements, good and bad, are absorbed into the bloodstream. The kidneys have the responsibility of filtering the impurities from the blood to be excreted from the body through urination.

The meal in this example placed an abundant acidic load on the kidneys. As a result, the body was forced to work very hard to extract the waste components posing a danger to the individual's overall health and received little compensation for its diligence in the form of nutrients.

A proper acid base balance is the foundation for maintaining health. Normal blood pH level ranges from 7.35 to 7.45. A pH rating is used to document the acid or alkaline level of a substance. In humans, blood, urine, saliva, and spinal fluid are measured for pH levels.

When the daily volume of food and beverages being ingested produces an acidic load on the kidneys, unwanted health issues begin to surface. The blood pH level registers below 7.35 and is referred to as acidosis.

The formula to maintain a proper acid base balance is 80/20. Consuming a diet of 80% alkaline and 20% acidic foods daily helps the body maintain a normal blood pH level. The Potential Renal Acid Load (PRAL) charts for individual food items and their associated potential renal acid or alkaline load are found in Chapter 6.

The Standard American Diet (SAD) is comprised of meat, dairy and bread products, poultry, farmed fish, and synthetic snacks and beverages. These items are acidic and place a significant and unnecessary burden on the kidneys.

As acidic food consumption continues, the kidneys become overwhelmed. The result is a decreased amount of waste being extracted from the blood and eliminated from the body.

Kidney stones can be expelled through urination as a natural progression from the kidney through the ureter to the bladder and finally the urethra. Larger stones can be broken into smaller pieces through a medical procedure called lithotripsy for easier, faster expulsion. These smaller pieces can then exit the body via urination. For very large stones, surgery may be required.

Calcium oxalate, cystine, and uric acid stones are formed in acidic urine.[1]

URIC ACID

Uric acid is a major contributor to the creation of kidney stones. Persons suffering from stones often experience the symptoms of gout, high blood pressure, and diabetes as well. These dangerous health conditions are fueled by similar eating habits and lifestyles.

Learning the process of uric acid development provides a framework for understanding the basis of stone formation. When animal protein is consumed, a special digestive enzyme, called pepsin, must enter the stomach to break down the heavy proteins. The deconstructed animal proteins are metabolized by the liver into amino acid chains for the body to utilize. This metabolic action produces ammonia, which is deadly to the body. The liver must re-metabolize this toxic ammonia byproduct. As a result of this process, uric acid is produced. Hence, restricted animal protein ingestion limits uric acid production and results in fewer impurities traveling to the kidneys. Uric acid serves as a foundation for kidney stone construction.

An article in the *European Journal of Epidemiology* reported the findings of a study that sought to identify an association between diet and kidney stone risk. There were 51,336 participants with a wide range of diets. The findings stated:

High intakes of fresh fruit, fiber from wholegrain cereals and magnesium were also associated with a lower risk of kidney stone formation. A high intake of zinc was associated with a higher risk. In conclusion, vegetarians have a lower risk of developing kidney stones compared with those who eat a high meat diet. This information may be important to advise the public about prevention of kidney stone formation.[2]

While high protein, low carbohydrate diets are being promoted as the healthiest weight loss programs available, it is difficult to find any clinical research to support eating animal flesh, poultry or fish three meals a day. This is one of the reasons why people get sick after following these high animal protein diets. These diets foster high cholesterol, osteoporosis, cardiovascular disease and, ultimately, kidney disease as well as elevate the risk of forming cancer.

Commercial meat products in the United States are contaminated with many chemicals. Some additives are considered so dangerous that many countries will not accept US beef, chicken, turkey, pork and farmed fish.[3,4] If these food products are part of your daily routine, then this information may be crucial for saving your life! US meats are banned in other countries for these reasons:

Arsenic. Although it is well known that arsenic is a noted carcinogen, it is widely used in commercial chicken feed to help kill parasites.

Beef. Cows can be fed synthetic growth hormones, antibiotics, steroids, and other chemicals generally added to commercial cattle feed. Some hormones and chemicals can be detected in the meat after slaughter and are linked to a variety of health issues.

Beef, chicken, pork, and turkey. These products are banned if the use of a food additive, Ractopamine, is identified. While it has not been proven to cause cancer, it is linked to increased heart rate and anxiousness.

Farmed fish. These fish are raised in an unnatural environment ingesting grains, chemicals, antibiotics, and drugs to restore their irregular color. They contain fewer nutrients and flavor due to their unnatural diet and living conditions. The drugs and other chemicals used in farm-raised fish have been proven to contribute to disease.

The list of chemicals and other additives in US meats is extensive! When eating commercial meats, the label does not list the undesirable components fed to and injected into the live animal nor the ones inserted in the meat, poultry, or fish after slaughter to retard oxidation, deterioration, and add color. Regardless of the words on the label, the liver and kidneys must manage the unlisted ingredients.

Is any meat safe? Yes. A grass-fed cow in the backyard, slaughtered by its owner, does not contain the hundreds of additives of commercially raised cows. Consuming red meat once a week from a homegrown source is very different from consuming commercial meat. The same is true for pastured chickens, turkeys, wild-caught fish, venison, elk, etc. A serving size of flesh, poultry, or fish is 4-6 ounces, but US restaurants offer larger sizes as normal portions.

Expiration dates. Food for thought: If a grass-fed cow from Jenny, the neighbor next door, is slaughtered on Saturday morning, and she brings two fresh steaks to your house, how long would you allow the steaks to sit in the refrigerator until you considered them too old to prepare? Three days or maybe five? The challenging part of commercial meat processing is keeping it from rotting after slaughter and still looking good enough to sell on a grocery shelf. To make that happen, chemicals must be added. While most people would not feel safe preparing a fresh steak after it remains in the refrigerator for five days or more, they are perfectly fine with buying one from the grocery market with an expiration date two weeks or longer from the date they purchase it.

Chemicals. Just because they are in a product does not mean they are safe. Many of the food additives Americans ingest are banned in other countries and rightfully so.[5]

When discussing this subject, it is interesting to hear what others believe about meat consumption and its heritage. Some express the idea that our forefathers only ate meat, and thus we should eat lots of meat as well. Nevertheless, such claims are not fact and are so far from the truth.

Our forefathers did eat meat, but it was not the only item on their dinner plate. It was, however, from a real animal unspoiled by chemicals, steroids, antibiotics, hormones, and toxic waste.

A wild boar hunted in the woods is an animal that provides meat. A commercial pig is raised in a confined area, fed manmade synthesized food, drugged, killed, and then marketed to you as *meat*. These two animals are not remotely the same.

A recent study found…

The consumption of beef dropped nearly 20% between 2004 and 2015 in the United States.[6]

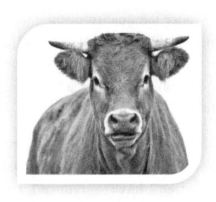

The high protein diet craze sounds great and can work if it is done correctly for a short period of time, but the long-term consequences of it are significant. Likewise, eating fast food burgers without the bread, frying up bacon and eggs every morning, or regularly consuming farmed fish is not a healthy diet. It is kidney damage in disguise.

If you are a carnivore, acknowledging the role that meat products play in uric acid accretion and kidney stone development must sound like a nightmare! Yet, there are ways to approach a healthier diet and still have some meat.

1. Breakfast: To save your kidneys and prevent stone formation, you can choose some berries or oatmeal, make a vegetable and fruit smoothie, opt for organic cereal. It is easier to eliminate meat from a breakfast meal than lunch or dinner for most people. Then, drink a full glass of water before going to work.
2. Lunch: Find somewhere to make your own salad or make one at home. Choose fruits and vegetables, beans, nuts, seeds, mushrooms, artichokes, and small portions of grains. Limit the salad dressing and pre-made pasta salads as they contain a high percentage of synthetic and chemical ingredients. Drink a full glass of water twenty minutes before eating.
3. Dinner: Now you can have some meat if you want it. You may want to consider the quality of the meat you choose. A fresh steak from a local butcher versus a fast-food rubbish patty. Eat vegetables with your meat in lieu of bread or starch options for proper food combining. Drink a full glass of water 20 minutes before eating.

The distressing truth is that the food you are paying a very high price to purchase is helping to form very painful kidney stones. Vegans and vegetarians have a reduced rate of kidney stones compared to meat-eaters. The major reason vegans and vegetarians ever develop kidney stones is that they were formed from eating meat before they adopted a non-meat diet.

When it comes to meat and uric acid, unfortunately, there is no way around it. The body performs digestion and elimination tasks based upon its own set of regulations. Uric acid is a byproduct of metabolizing animal protein. To reduce uric acid and limit the risk of kidney stones, the quality of the meat choices and how much meat is consumed requires some consideration.

DEHYDRATION

Water is a basic requirement for sustaining life. It effects all functions in the body from swallowing to pumping your heart and helping you think.

Here is the water content of:

Lungs	83%
Kidneys and muscles	79%
Brain and heart	73%
Skin	64%
Bones	31%[7]

The water content of muscles and bones is age-related. Younger bones require more water.

A person can survive for three days without water and three weeks without food. Nearly every person on earth has experienced some type of dehydration symptom. It could be a headache or muscle cramp. Without appropriate amounts of water, the kidneys cannot operate properly. As the water content list above conveys, kidneys require more water to function than the brain and heart.

Pure, clean water helps to keep them healthy so they can:

1. Filter waste and toxins from the blood
2. Regulate minerals in the blood
3. Maintain the body's fluid balance
4. Make hormones:
a. Renin - To regulate blood pressure
b. Erythropoietin (EPO) - To produce red blood cells via bone marrow
5. Consistently help clear toxins from the kidneys

Kidneys are the extraordinary heroes working hard every millisecond to save your life! Water is extracted from all forms of food and drink.

When consuming manmade, synthetic, dry, no-nutritional-value junk foods with coffee, energy drinks, soda, and other toxic beverages, dehydration follows. The additives in the beverages alone cannot produce enough hydration to absorb the impact of the low water content food or snack choices.

Manufactured products such as potato, corn, and tortilla chips, crackers, popcorn, granola bars, and rice cakes contain very low water content. They normally average less than 5% water content.

Nuts range from 5% to 15% water content:[8]

Pecans	5%	Walnuts	5%
Almonds	6%	Brazil	7%
Peanuts	7%	Pistachio	7%
Cashew	8%	Hazelnut	15%
Macadamia	15%		

A slice of watermelon is 92% water content. All fruits and vegetables contain water packed with valuable nutrients. Celery tops the list with 95% water content, vitamins, minerals, antioxidants, alkalinity, and zero calories. In addition, celery is proven to help flush toxins from the body.

This information about water content in food helps explain why dehydration becomes such an issue in our convenient, pre-packaged food and drink culture.

The "I Dare You to Be Honest with Yourself" List

How many ounces do you drink in a day?

Water	Coffee	Tea
Soda	Energy Drinks	Juice
Beer	Wine	Spirits
Milk	Kombucha	Kiefer
Soup Broth	Hot Chocolate	Smoothies

This mental exercise helps you realize how many total ounces of liquids you are consuming that contain toxins versus the total ounces of water to help the kidneys do their job effectively for your better health.

The secret to maintaining health and drinking something other than water is balance. For example, drinking a glass of wine will not create a severe negative impact on the kidneys if appropriate amounts of water are being consumed before and after the wine.

Morning tea or coffee are no problem when drinking water throughout the day and adding some fresh fruits and vegetables.

MYTHS ABOUT WATER CONSUMPTION

Hydrates if made of water

Let's use coffee as an example. It is made with water and ground coffee beans. Two ingredients. The water is hydrating, and the caffeine in the coffee beans creates minimal dehydration. Plain black coffee in moderation is okay. However, drinking coffee with sugar, creamer, whipped cream, and flavored oils creates dehydration. It is the additives that pose an issue, not the coffee itself.

Caffeine, manmade sugars, and other ingredients must be filtered from the blood because they are waste rather than nutrients. The water-based beverage serves as a method to carry the toxins into and through the body.

If it is made of water, there is some level of hydration associated with the beverage. When the beverage is predominately synthetic and chemical components, it becomes more detrimental to kidney health than what the minimal hydration level offers.

Causes bloating.

Water is absorbed through the stomach approximately twenty minutes after you drink it. Water does not cause bloating on its own. The reason people feel bloated after drinking water is due to other factors.

One cause of bloating is the level of sodium in the body is too high because of dehydration. Drinking more water when you feel bloated will reduce the sodium, thus reducing the amount of fluid being retained. We need sodium to survive. Processed foods contain higher sodium content than often recognized. Thus, it is important to maintain a healthy sodium to water ratio.

A second cause of bloating is that certain vitamin and mineral levels are insufficient to adequately eliminate excess fluids. When magnesium, potassium, vitamin C, or the B vitamins are low, then water retention occurs. These vitamins and minerals are required for optimum kidney function. Eating fresh fruits and vegetables high in these nutrients can quickly relieve bloating.

Drink only when thirsty.

This myth has dangerous possibilities! If you are sweating in high heat, the body must do everything to protect itself. By the time you feel dizziness and start experiencing heat rash and thirst, it may be too late to arrest that level of dehydration and electrolyte loss without medical attention. This situation is called heat stroke.

We are living in a land of manmade synthetic foods and drinks. We are human beings with basic needs. We require appropriate amounts of pure water for proper operation of all our elaborate, incredible body systems. This myth could cost you your life.

Drink pure water throughout the day. It will keep you hydrated and help flush out the toxins that cause kidney stones. Soda and other synthetic beverages do not qualify as acceptable replacements for water.

According to a study by the Centers for Disease Control and Prevention:

- 43% of adults drink less than four cups of water daily
- 36% drink one to three cups
- 7% drink none

Eight glasses a day.

Drink eight glasses of water a day. This is a guideline to help maintain hydration. There are really no hard and fast rules for water consumption except this one: monitor the color of your urine.

If it is dark in color or has an odor, drinking eight glasses of water may be your best approach. Dark urine is a sign of dehydration and high levels of toxic waste. Prescription medications, artificially colored snacks, excess meat, and fast food consumption, illegal drugs, combined with a diet low in fresh fruits and vegetables, can generate this situation. Drink enough water daily until urine is very pale yellow to nearly clear. The kidneys are the heroes that save your life. Give them enough pure, clean water to do their job.

Sports drinks.

Sports drinks are designed to replace electrolytes lost during intense exercise or extreme heat. Many sports drinks contain sugar, artificial colors, flavors, and additives. Pure water is a better choice if you are not participating in heavy physical activity or dealing with extreme heat conditions.

Sodium, potassium, calcium, magnesium, phosphorus, and chloride are examples of electrolytes essential for sustaining life. These vitamins and minerals help balance fluids and control bodily functions. Eating fresh fruits and vegetables daily will provide you with sufficient amounts of these nutrients.

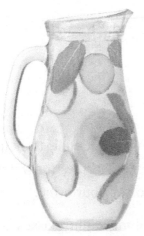

Persons performing physical labor tasks in all types of weather outdoors, those exposed to high temperature jobs indoors, first responders enduring intense heat situations, utility workers, construction workers, road crews and farmers, are more likely to require electrolyte drinks than others. Many of these occupations are trained to alternate between water and electrolyte drinks.

Making a refreshing electrolyte drink can be fun and easy. Slice lemon, lime, orange, or cucumber and add a small pinch of sea salt. Frozen strawberries, raspberries, or sprigs of fresh herbs from the garden are tasty additions to water.

Water is the fountain of youth. It helps restore and hydrate every cell in the body and significantly reduces your risk of kidney stone formation. Sports drinks are expensive, and some ingredients can impair health.

MEDICATIONS

Medications come with side effects. Some of them have more damaging effects on kidneys than others. A kidney stone is an indication that future, possibly severe kidney conditions that could surface unless changes are made to promote kidney health.

Prescription medications in the United States are viewed by the population as generally safe. The opioid crisis illuminated not only the dangers of specific medications but how easy it was to obtain these highly addictive and damaging pills.

Not all medications are addictive; however, all medications do have a negative impact on good health. When you are prescribed a medication to treat a symptom, the decline of your health continues. Better health begins with identifying the cause and correcting it.

Below is a list of the medication categories recognized for contributing to kidney stone formation. Not every prescription medication in the category is as damaging as another. Please review your medication to see if kidney stones or kidney damage are a listed side effect.

Antacid	Antibiotic	Anticonvulsant
Antifungal	Antiviral	Anxiety
Chemotherapy	Cholesterol	Contrast dyes
Decongestant	Depression	Diabetes
Diuretics	H2 Blockers	HIV/AIDS
Hypertension	Migraine	Pain Relief
Seizure	Steroid	Ulcer

Proton Pump Inhibitor

With most prescription medications, there are benefits and side effects. For many, the benefits may be perceived to outweigh the harm. Stones are a sign that your kidneys are confronting undue stress and difficulty. Since multiple factors contribute to their formation, determining if the prescription you are taking is the best choice within the medication category may be a starting point to eliminating a known factor contributing to stone formation and the probability of kidney disease.

Once you have identified the underlying issue, plan to address the cause of the condition. If the medication is for high blood pressure, reduce high sodium processed foods. Diabetes, gastrointestinal disorders, acid reflux, headaches, and cholesterol, for example, can be addressed through diet choices and hydration. Junk foods are not really food and can wreak havoc on good health and the wallet. Clean eating can help reduce the need for prescription medications, reduce the amount of money spent on doctor's visits, blood tests, and medicine, promote longevity, and best of all, decrease the chances of kidney stones.

A Mayo Clinic study reveals...

Among Americans, 70% are taking at least one prescription medication and 20% are taking five or more medically prescribed drugs.[10]

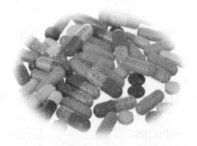

INFLAMMATORY BOWEL DISEASE

"All disease begins in the gut."

Regarded as the father of medicine, Hippocrates made this statement nearly 2400 years ago.

Inflammatory Bowel Disease (IBD) refers to health conditions arising when the gastrointestinal tract is chronically inflamed. Crohn's disease and ulcerative colitis are generally consolidated under the umbrella of IBD.

A diet high in processed foods and animal protein, farmed fish, prescription and over-the-counter medications, illegal drugs, smoking, vaping, and lifestyle habits contribute to IBD.

Likewise, a lack of water and nutritious foods plays a predominant role in irritating the colon.

Persons diagnosed with IBD have a 38% chance of developing kidney stones.[11] This statistic from 2013 is a frightening announcement. Imagine what the percentage might be today with the alarming increases in IBD and kidney stone disease.

Many IBD conditions can be remedied and reversed with dietary and habit changes. The same eating habits associated with IBD and other compromised intestinal conditions are the same habits that contribute to the highest percentage of kidney stones.

Eliminating or significantly reducing the foods and drinks associated with declining health issues will further limit IBD conditions and help hinder the looming threat of developing kidney stones.

The foods you choose to eat either promote health or diminish it. You didn't get to this point overnight. Take baby steps. Begin with eliminating a fast food meal. Trade the breakfast sandwich for an organic piece of fruit and take some of your favorite raw vegetables for a mid-morning snack. Essentially, you just traded toxic, man-altered foods for highly nutritious, health-promoting, wholesome and natural food. Settle into this new routine, then reduce soda and replace it with water. Changing habits does not have to be difficult.

Keep it simple. Drink more water and less processed beverages. Eat more fruits and vegetables and less processed foods. Choose a variety of fruits and vegetables that you enjoy. Try something new on occasion. Wholesome nutrition and proper hydration will reward you with better overall health.

The High Price of a Kidney Stone . . .

Urine tests, blood tests, CT scans, MRIs, sonograms, physician and specialist visits, medications, stone analysis, urgent care, and emergency room charges can add up to thousands of dollars. For the person with very limited or no insurance, a kidney stone may cost more than an automobile or rent for a year!

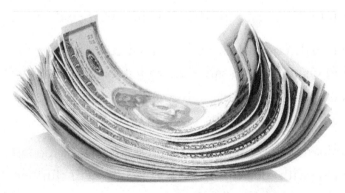

DIABETES

There are a variety of factors associated with diabetes and forming kidney stones. Several of those contributors were listed previously: uric acid, dehydration, and medications.

In the US, 43% of persons seeking medical attention for kidney stones have previously been diagnosed with type 2 diabetes mellitus (T2DM).[12]

The outstanding correlation between kidney stones and diabetes is dietary intake. Persons with T2DM take medication to help lower blood glucose levels without being properly instructed on how the body metabolizes food.

Diabetics typically believe their condition is inherited. This is an untrue statement for ninety five percent of diabetes diagnoses.

Unless you were born with diabetes, have a physical injury to the pancreas, or sustained damage to the pancreas through a virus or an illness, a diabetes diagnosis can be reversed through dietary changes.

This incredible statement from Yuval Noah Harari in the book *Homo Deus: A History of Tomorrow,* illustrates these facts better than any words I've ever read:

> In 2012 about 56 million people died throughout the world; 620,000 of them died due to human violence (war killed 120,000 people, and crime killed another 500,000). In contrast, 800,000 committed suicide, and 1.5 million died of diabetes. Sugar is now more dangerous than gunpowder. (15)[13]

Having diabetes and kidney stones tells a critical health story. The body is already struggling to process the individual's daily food and drink choices. Without substantial positive changes in diet, more complex health conditions are on the horizon.

Ninety-five percent of Americans choose to remain diabetic for two major reasons. One, they are addicted to the foods they love.

Two, they do not have access to truthful education about foods and nutrition. These manmade, addictive snacks and food pretenders are deliberately laden with additives to help create that addiction.

After delivering a speech about the impending shortage of insulin shots and diabetes medications by the year 2030, some people formed a line to ask for personal insight concerning their health situation. A mild-mannered gentleman said this to me, "I know bread is supposed to be bad for you, but as a Christian, I cannot give it up because Jesus fed it to the masses. How can you say with such assurance that bread promotes diabetes? Is it because you are not a Christian?"

This was a correlation to the past I had not heard before. I explained that the bread in the era of Jesus was unleavened, non-GMO, contained no additives, preservatives, artificial ingredients, and was usually eaten alone. Furthermore, people walked, did manual labor daily, and expended energy, thus requiring carbohydrate consumption.

Diabetes is not created by bread alone. Bread-type products are a standard option for American meal combinations or snacks. Sandwiches, pizza, wraps, pasta, bakery items, desserts, crackers, and pretzels are just a few examples.

These items metabolize into blood glucose. Diabetes would not be as pervasive if these items were consumed based upon the serving size and choosing only one bread product per day.

Having a T2DM diagnosis is not a life sentence. People have the power to alter their diet and invest in recovering their health. This is where the education piece comes into play.

When T2DM is being managed, not corrected, but managed by medication, some assume it is their only option. Popping a pill daily to help control blood glucose levels becomes a way of life. Since the underlying cause of the condition was not addressed with education and appropriate dietary changes, the next health issue arises. Kidney stones and heart disease are serious future health concerns for diabetics.

Imagine learning years after the fact that with proper dietary education, the hardship of diabetes, kidney stones, and the ensuing heart condition could have been averted. All the money spent on medications, appointments, blood tests, medical supplies, and so on, would be in your bank account or spent on your hopes and dreams.

Consistent consumption of processed foods diminishes health. With T2DM comes a 43% or higher chance of forming kidney stones and developing other health complications. Consuming a more nutritious diet high in fresh fruits and vegetables is highly encouraged.

A serving size of most fruits contains less sugar and carbohydrates than one slice of bread. If a diabetic can eat bread and crackers, then they can eat fruit. Fruits are packed with vitamins and minerals, made by nature, and the body can recognize and easily assimilate their nutrients.

By contrast, breads and crackers are not produced in nature. They do turn into blood glucose, just like fruit, but contain far less nutritional value.

HEARTBURN, REFLUX, INDIGESTION

Only in the United States do people sincerely believe that at some point in their life, they will develop excess stomach acid for no real reason. This is a concocted misrepresentation of bodily functions and is not true.

The Standard American Diet (SAD) is filled with sodium, fats, grease, cholesterol, synthetic components, and is a disaster for the body to digest and metabolize into usable nutrients.

Heartburn, indigestion, and acid reflux are symptoms of multiple causes. The primary issue to consider here is overeating. The size of your fist represents the size your stomach is supposed to be when empty. When eating a double cheeseburger, French fries, and drinking a 20-ounce soda, the stomach becomes stuffed beyond capacity and stretches. It will take approximately 10 hours to digest this combination. It is more food than can comfortably be accommodated by the digestive system, especially if an earlier meal has not yet been fully digested. To ease this type of discomfort, eat smaller meals and snack on fresh fruits and vegetables throughout the day.

Other major causes of these digestive issues are smoking, alcohol consumption, obesity, pregnancy, carbonated beverages, certain health conditions, and medications.

Americans spend more than $2 billion dollars a year on prescription and over-the-counter antacid products! But these products come with serious side effects.

The American Society of Nephrology states that,

Certain medications commonly used to treat heartburn, acid reflux, and ulcers can have damaging effects on the kidneys.[16]

Medications known as PPIs increase the risk of kidney stones by 12% and H2 blockers create a 13% higher risk of having a kidney stone.[16]

By taking steps to stop the cause, you can dramatically decrease your risk of developing kidney stones.

- Fully chew food before swallowing it
- Eat slowly
- Choose wholesome foods versus fried or fatty ones
- Drink more water than manmade beverages
- Tomato-based red sauces often contribute to digestive upset because many tomatoes are peeled with lye instead of steam. If this is true for you, remove them from your diet to see if the reflux, heartburn, and indigestion subside without the help of medications or switch to an organic tomato sauce option.

CALCIUM OXALATE STONES

Calcium oxalate stones are the most documented type and seemingly the most difficult to understand. Here's why.

The information about their formation is misunderstood and largely publicized incorrectly. For example: calcium oxalate stones are "supposedly" caused by spinach and other high oxalate containing vegetables. *This statement is entirely false*. Let's think about that for a minute.

Persons that *rarely* eat spinach, asparagus or drink loose leaf black or green teas, are instructed to avoid these items because they are the major contributors to this form of kidney stone. How can that be true? If you do not eat spinach, how can it help to form a kidney stone inside your body? It cannot.

Persons with kidney stones documented as being calcium oxalate based often report an insignificant consumption of any high oxalate vegetables. The concentration of calcium oxalate and/or calcium phosphate is associated with multiple health complications and lifestyle choices, not consuming certain vegetables and teas. A registered dietician and researcher from the University of Wisconsin-Madison Department of Urology states:

The foods that are highest in oxalate are also high in fiber, magnesium, potassium, and phytate. These are actually stone inhibitors. Moreover, studies show that when you reduce oxalate, you reduce your fiber intake. That can lead to constipation and other bowel issues. In general, we're trying to help people eat a healthy, balanced diet.[17]

The real cause of calcium oxalate stones is the intake of highly processed foods. These foods complicate the nutrient assimilation function in the colon. The corrupted forms of calcium from processed foods bind with oxalates that the body produces to protect itself in the intestines. This process derails normal calcium absorption.

Another intricate issue arises when the lack of appropriate amounts of wholesome, natural forms of calcium are not being consumed. Calcium is required for healthy nerve function, muscle contractions, steady heart rhythms, healthy bones and teeth. Calcium must bond with protein molecules and is assisted by magnesium and vitamin D, for superior absorption.

Eating a fast-food cheeseburger, French fries, and drinking a soda has a higher contribution to kidney stone formation than any amount of high oxalate fruits and vegetables. The contaminants in fast-food create dehydration, impair all functions of the digestive system, and when oxalates are needed, the body creates them on its own.

The combination of corrupt calcium sources being ingested with foodstuffs containing phosphorus creates an environment conducive for a kidney-stone-making-jubilee. Our culinary delights are improperly combined for human digestion and nutrient orientation.

A combination of meat, bread, and cheese essentially violates every natural rule for human food consumption. There is no sandwich in nature, unfortunately. They are delicious but inflict pandemonium on kidney function.

Acidosis is the major reason for any type of kidney stone. In calcium-based stones, the body's compromised ability to absorb calcium through the blood creates the opportunity for calcium and oxalates to accumulate in the kidneys. Persons consuming a diet low in fresh fruits and vegetables often experience acidosis. When blood and urine drop below 7.35 pH level, it is considered acidic and unable to function at an optimal level. Chronic acidosis occurs at a 6.5 pH level or below. Alkalinity occurs at a 7.4 pH level.

Chronic intestinal issues inhibit proper calcium absorption.

Calcium requires nutrients to be present in the blood to provide the highest level of absorption. Magnesium, vitamin D, vitamin C, and vitamin K help promote calcium assimilation. Certain medications interfere with vitamin D activity. Therefore, it is not available to assist with calcium absorption.

Carbonated water, soda, and some energy drinks can contain phosphoric acid, which interferes with proper calcium uptake and helps create an environment for kidney stone formation. When consuming these drinks daily, the risk of creating a stone becomes increasingly prevalent.

The contribution to calcium oxalate and calcium phosphate stones from processed meats, seafood, and farmed fish is extraordinary. The list includes:

- bacon, sausage – pork or turkey
- salami, pepperoni, deli meats, hot dogs
- liver, other animal organs

- mussels, scallops, oysters
- shrimp, crab, lobster

Consuming these foods occasionally will not create a major health issue. Processed meats have become a basic part of the Standard American Diet (SAD) for many people. In 2015, the World Health Organization listed bacon, sausage, hot dogs, and salami as leading carcinogens.[18]

These processed meat items contain high amounts of contaminants that restrict vitamin and mineral absorption, create digestive issues, and are proven to cause colorectal cancer. They are listed beside plutonium, cigarettes, and asbestos as cancer-causing substances.

Excessive alcohol consumption and drug use, recreational and illegal, is proven to significantly contribute to stone formation. These items hinder the precise utilization of all nutrients, including calcium.

According to Dr. Veronique Desaulniers, persons taking calcium supplements regularly have higher incident rates of forming kidney stones. She also states that approximately 60% to 80% of oxalates are formed by the body.[19]

People search for a few things they can avoid to reduce the risk of stones when the answer is truly very simple. The body requires a balance of water and nutrients for optimum wellness. When food does not resemble anything produced in nature, it becomes difficult to sustain any level of good health. Think of it this way: An apple is an apple. A carrot is a carrot. Junk food is exactly that, junk food. The kidneys know the difference. They help keep humans alive when the basics of nutrition are purposefully ignored. Eat an apple instead of a breakfast bar. Try a fresh green salad in lieu of a fast-food lunch. Before long, your new choices will reward you with better health and reduce your risk of kidney stones.

Foods to eliminate:

Processed meats - bacon, sausage, hot dogs, salami

Fast food meats burgers, fried chicken, ham, pork barbeque

Energy drinks, soda, juice containing phosphoric acid

Farmed fish – all

Shellfish - Shrimp, crab, lobster, oysters

Seafood Mussels, clams, scallops, shark, mackerel, swordfish

Artificial sweeteners – all

Conventional dairy products

Non-dairy coffee creamer

High fructose corn syrup

Popcorn all

The list may seem overwhelming, but kidney stones are a symptom of more serious kidney disease lurking in your future unless you make some dietary changes. Choose one to eliminate each week. Start with soda or energy drinks. If you must have soda, drink less of it and more water, and find a soda without phosphoric acid. Then eliminate bacon. Then popcorn. Then fast foods . . .

Foods to add:

Drink a minimum of 48 ounces of water a day.

2 servings of fresh fruit, 4 servings of fresh vegetables daily.

If you must have dairy, please consider organic options

Conventional dairy milk, yogurt, and cheese contains unwanted by-products that can contribute to stones.

Organic spices add delicious flavor to any meal. Most spices aid in proper digestion and help reduce inflammation.

Learn to drink coffee black or with minimal creamer.

Eat ¼ cup of good grains daily: white, brown or wild rice, oatmeal, quinoa, millet, etc. Pastas, bread and bakery items do not qualify as a good grain. They are manmade.

Add organic raisins to a meal or snack. They are the most alkaline food on earth.

Oven-baked or roasted sweet potato. They are a good source of calcium and can help satisfy a sweet tooth.

Eat small portions of good sources of fat: olives, avocado, coconut, wild-caught salmon, tuna, and sardines.

Only eat animal protein once a day if you cannot live without it. Eat a 4 to 6 ounce portion of meat at the evening meal with vegetables (corn, potatoes, and peas are considered starches, not vegetables). Mixing animal protein with starch reduces the proper absorption of vitamins and minerals.

STRUVITE STONES

Struvite stones are less common and are created in a shorter period of time. Struvite is a composition of magnesium, ammonium, and phosphate minerals produced by bacteria in the upper urinary tract. These stones can occur in persons with urinary catheters, urinary tract infections or those predisposed to frequent bladder or kidney infections.

Other contributing factors include alcohol and narcotic drug use, prescription and over-the-counter medications, kidney, liver and bowel diseases, bleeding ulcers, and other more advanced health conditions.

Struvite stones account for approximately 10% to 15% of all kidney stones.[20] Because they are a result of bacteria, they are faster growing, can be much larger in size and sometimes, form branches. Ouch! Avoiding them requires consistent hydration, addressing and removing the cause for urinary tract infection (UTI), and maintaining clean eating habits.

For females, urinating shortly after sexual intercourse considerably reduces the probability of developing a UTI.

Another healthy routine is fully relieving the bladder when feeling the urge to urinate. Persons performing certain occupations are more likely to develop UTIs because they "hold it" due to extenuating circumstances.

Other UTI contributors are diabetes, obesity, poor hygiene, lack of mobility, a compromised immune system, and overall health deterioration. Hydration, good hygiene, and healthy eating habits significantly reduce the risk of struvite stones.

CHAPTER 4

THE TRUTH ABOUT ALCOHOL

When lecturing on any health subject, the story arises that someone's grandfather drank ten beers every day and never had kidney stones. Another audience member chimes in that their grandfather drank a pint of whiskey every day, and they did not have liver or kidney disease.

My first response is to thank them for sharing and then ask if their grandfather worked outside or in an office for most of their life. The response is: they worked outside.

No two people on earth ever have the exact same nutrient levels, experiences, or eating habits. However, these two gentlemen had four incredible commonalities.

One, they worked outside in the sunshine and maintained a healthy level of natural vitamin D, which is required for appropriate calcium uptake and liver health.

Two, they most likely drank lots of pure water throughout the day because they were exposed to the elements. Water in the heat, hot coffee or tea in the winter.

Three, their beer and whiskey, along with their food, was not genetically modified, nor was it laden with pesticides, artificial ingredients, and other toxins unfit for human consumption for most of their lives.

Four, when they sat down after working all day and ate their dinner or supper, many of these gentlemen did not spend the remainder of the evening grazing on snacks and manmade junk. For many men and women of this generation, food and snacks after the evening meal were considered gluttony. Alcoholic beverages were not usually served with meals. Wine was taken one hour before a meal. Food was given achance to digest before having a beer or whiskey later in the evening.

Consuming alcohol today has many differences from the past. The older guys and gals drink their whiskey straight or on ice. The idea of diluting a carefully distilled, high-quality whiskey was silly. The fact that they preferred straight whiskey over mixed drinks most likely extended their life and kidney health.

Sodas, in the United States, contain unsavory ingredients that lead to kidney stone formation. Beyond that, many people drink alcohol with their meals, which contains kidney stone forming, synthetic junk posing as food.

Excessive alcohol consumption creates kidney stones. Responsible alcohol intake does not. Here is the truth and the reason why.

Beer. If you are drinking beer every day and eating junk food, you *are* a candidate for kidney stones. It does not have anything to do with the beer alone. Dehydration and chemical contamination from synthetic foods is the problem. Beer is not a stand-alone issue for creating stones.

You may want to consider upgrading to bottles instead of cans to lessen unwanted toxins such as bisphenol A (BPA). It is a chemical used inside cans that leaches into the contents. BPA is known to cause numerous health conditions even at low doses. You may want to find out if your favorite beer choices are BPA-free. Toxins are acidic and help create an environment for kidney stone formation.

Bottom line: Minimal consumption of beer itself does not cause kidney stones. Alcohol, of any kind, can trigger dehydration, which causes reduced kidney function, and ultimately, helps create kidney stones. Use this rule and having a beer will be less threatening to the kidneys. Drink a beer then drink some water.

Wine. Drinking red wine is associated with many wonderful health benefits, especially when it is not contaminated with GMOs, pesticides, artificial ingredients, and fillers.

For red wines, such as merlot, cabernet sauvignon, or cabernet franc, extraordinary health benefits can be derived when consumed responsibly. Wines are rich in antioxidants, polyphenols, minerals, and some vitamins. White wines contain the same benefits at lower levels.

At lectures, I hear the question asking, "Why do I always get a headache when drinking red wine, and how does it cause kidney stones?" Great question!

You are more likely to experience a headache after drinking red wine when you are sipping it while:

- eating iron-rich foods
- enjoying sugary desserts or chocolate
- taking medication
- dehydrated
- menstruating
- crying

Without the involvement of wine, dehydration, crying, menstruation, and medications can cause headaches. Some people interpret the headache after consuming wine to mean that wine is not good for them.

The grapes used to make the wine are incredibly rich in iron. When you pair a glass or two of red wine with iron-rich foods, such as a steak or spinach salad, a massive headache may erupt later if you are not properly hydrated.

There are 75 to 100 grapes in one glass of wine. Once the grapes are fermented, the vitamin and mineral composition does not remain the same as raw grapes. It becomes a concentrated source of pesticides, residues, sulfites, iron, minerals, vitamins, antioxidants and polyphenols. This combination generates intense cellular warriors to help you or hurt you depending upon the status of your body at that moment.

Iron can inhibit the absorption of calcium if it enters the body from two separate sources. Iron from wine and calcium from strawberries, for example. The iron inhibits the absorption of calcium and vice versa. In many cultures, it is customary to drink wine one hour before the meal; not with the meal. This tradition honors the natural rules of digestion. Within 20 minutes of finishing the wine, the usable nutrients are absorbed. The stomach is now ready for the next course, fruits or salad.

Bottom line: One glass of wine alone does not cause kidney stones when you are properly hydrated.

Whiskey or Vodka: Due to the higher content of ethanol, these alcoholic drinks can impair all functions of the body when consumed in excess. However, when consuming one jigger of whiskey or vodka, the outcome is equivalent to beer or wine. It is what the whiskey or vodka is being consumed *with* that can construct an environment for the creation of kidney stones. Just like wine, straight spirits are less likely to impact kidney stones development when consumed an hour prior to a meal or hours after a meal rather than during a meal or combined with other beverages.

Bottom line: Spirits alone do not create kidney stones if the person is properly hydrated and having one drink that is not combined with a sugary juice or soda. Alcohol creates dehydration, which causes reduced kidney function, and can contribute to stones especially when consumed in excess.

Partaking of Libations:

People drink alcoholic beverages for many reasons. It tastes good to them. It is a social thing. A glass of wine before dinner. A jigger of scotch before bed.

There is a huge difference between consuming one drink responsibly and binge drinking on Friday and Saturday nights or any time of the day. Intoxication creates an environment with multiple complications. Dehydration is the most prominent issue often accompanied by headache and hangover. To remedy the uncomfortable body aches, pain relievers are taken to address the headache and other over the counter aids are used for nausea and lack of energy.

To understand stone formation, we must first understand our bodies as a whole unit. It is not one thing, like alcohol, that causes kidney stones. Our bodies survive on nutrition. When the foodstuffs we are cramming into our bodies do not meet any type of natural quality standards, bad outcomes can happen for the whole body, not just kidneys. We have been conditioned to look for a definitive answer about each item we eat or drink rather than obtaining a full picture of kidney function and stone development.

An article titled, *Soda and Other Beverages and the Risk of Kidney Stones*, concludes that:

> Consumption of sugar-sweetened soda and punch is associated with a higher risk of stone formation, whereas consumption of coffee, tea, beer, wine, and orange juice is associated with a lower risk.[1]

Coffee, tea, beer, wine and orange juice are made from nature. Coffee beans and oranges come from trees. Tea leaves from plants. Wine from fruit of the vines. Both beer and wine are fermented and offer probiotics and nutrients. Soda and energy drinks cannot meet any of these standards. They are manmade disasters for the kidneys.

If you want to drink a beer, no problem. You want a glass of wine before dinner or do a shot to celebrate, do it. During these occasions, just say no to the animal protein and make sure you drink some water to stay hydrated. One drink is not a health disaster. It is the lack of nutrients from food choices coupled with dehydration that causes many health issues, as well as kidney stones.

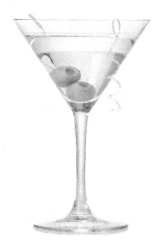

I drink too much.
The last time I gave a urine sample,
it have an olive in it.

- Rodney Dangerfield[2]

CHAPTER 5

STONE FORMATION MYTHS

GENETICS

I'm sorry. The parental gene pool is not to blame for nearly 80% of kidney stone issues. This statement is only true if you have one rare kidney stone disease, cystinuria. The remaining stones are formed through diet, consistent dehydration or bacterial infection. I apologized because someone has led many people to believe a falsehood about the genetic role associated with kidney stones.

If stones were truly inherited, why would people stop having this issue once they switched to more wholesome, natural foods?

The answer is remarkably straightforward. It is eating habits that are 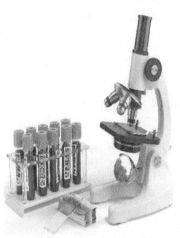 inherited. Very frequently, eating habits are repeated by the next generation. Foods eaten as children or teens may have contributed to the stone, but genetics did not create it.

Scientific reports do state that kidney stones are created in individuals with similar habits. The findings do not report genetic transfer of kidney stone genes (unless cystinuria). Science concludes that without having cystinuria, the only familial incidence of stones that can be traced or observed with any accuracy is food consumption and lifestyle habits.

TEA

I once witnessed a medical doctor stating that tea caused kidney stones. Slightly taken aback, I asked what kind of tea. Was it black, green, herbal? He responded by saying it was all tea. No wonder myths are created!

Loose-leaf green tea is the most studied plant on earth. It is scientifically proven to help prevent and fight certain types of cancer, lower risks of liver, kidney, and heart disease, promote health at all levels, and minimize the risk of dementia.

If green tea caused kidney stones, how would anyone in certain countries where most of their population drinks four to six cups of loose leaf tea daily ever get out of bed? Let's think about that. Kidney stones are painful. If tea truly caused kidney stones, it would disable entire countries!

Tea contains polyphenols and superb antioxidants that serve as stone inhibitors. Drinking real, loose leaf tea is the fastest way to better health. It helps fortify every cell in the body.

Artificially tea flavored, manmade crystals that dissolve in water may contribute to stones. Real tea leaves do not dissolve. Bottled sweet tea with high fructose corn syrup may cause stones also. While these beverages are called "tea," they contain synthetic ingredients, and are not the same as loose leaf tea. It would be like stating that a sports car and a van are the same because they are both automobiles.

I was always brought up to have a cup of tea at halfway up a rock face. --Bear Grylls

HIGH CALCIUM FOODS

Avoiding high calcium foods can threaten your overall health. The real reason for calcium oxalate or calcium phosphate stones is the body's inability to remove the excess impurities from the kidneys due to dehydration and lack of vital nutrients. Wholesome sources of calcium are essential for your body to operate. Calcium supplements are not natural and can contribute to stone formation. Fresh fruits and vegetables rank at the top of the chart for wholesome sources of digestible, usable forms of calcium.

When the body does not have enough calcium to help the organs perform their purpose, the blood will extract calcium from the bones to help all of the body's systems function.

Eating high calcium foods *does not* cause kidney stones even though it is widely printed online. Yes. **I am stating that all those articles are incorrect**. No worries. I can prove it.

The most impressive example of calcium oxalate kidney stone formation is that associated with astronauts. While in space, they consume less water, eat high sodium rations, rarely eat fresh produce, and experience limited resistance exercise.

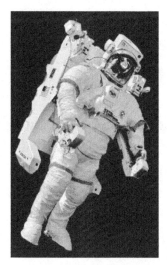

Astronauts leave Earth in extraordinarily good health, but experience bone loss in space. The body extracts calcium from the bones due to insufficient wholesome sources of this essential nutrient available during the mission. According to the National Aeronautics and Space Administration (NASA), kidney stones have been reported in excess of 30 times by astronaut's postflight.

[1] *Figure 1 Photo by Christian Wagner, Unsplash.com*

The word "calcium oxalate" is the term associated with the predominate substance combinations identified in a kidney stone. For calcium to properly be absorbed and utilized in the bloodstream, it binds with a protein molecule. The following information is listed on the United States Department of Health & Human Services, National Institutes of Health, Office of Dietary Supplements website:

Most kidney stones are rich in calcium oxalate. Some studies have found that higher intakes of calcium from dietary supplements are linked to a greater risk of kidney stones, especially among older adults. But **calcium from foods does not appear to cause kidney stones.** For most people, other factors (such as not drinking enough fluids) probably have a larger effect on the risk of kidney stones than calcium intake.[2]

I describe supplements this way. It does not matter if you swallow them or toss them in your backyard, you will receive the same amount of usable calcium. Most brands of supplements are synthetic, worthless, and help create stones.

Spinach, kale, rhubarb, loose leaf tea, nuts, okra, collard greens, and broccoli offer a variety of vital nutrients. The calcium and oxalates in these foods serve your body as stone inhibitors. They do not act as a detriment.

Stones form because of other factors, not because of calcium. Dehydration, eating more processed foods than fresh fruits and vegetables, consuming U.S. meats, smoking, vaping, consuming excessive alcohol, and a huge list of other unhealthy habits cause calcium oxalate stones. These lifestyle factors inhibit kidney function, thus disallowing the ability to fully void toxic, unusable ingested elements.

High calcium fruits and vegetables are the path to no more kidney stones. Want more proof? Just ask the person who passed a kidney stone and was told it is calcium oxalate stone how much spinach, figs, and oranges they eat? When they tell you they do not eat those foods, then ask the next person. After hearing countless stories from people you know with calcium oxalate stones that do not eat any measurable quantities of beets, kale, spinach, almonds, and so on, it can serve as your own little research project to be convinced that spinach is good for you.

Here are some wholesome forms of calcium:

- Fresh fruits and vegetables.
- Wild-caught salmon, tuna, sardines
- Raw nuts, seeds, and cacao nibs
- White beans, lentils, black-eyed peas
- Good grains
- All local grass-fed meats

Please keep in mind that processed foods contain corrupt forms of calcium and sodium.

HIGH FAT DIET

A diet high in animal fat "supposedly" reverses kidney disease and reduces kidney stones according to some blogs and unsubstantiated claims. This statement is so horrifically misinterpreted, it is terrifying. I met a woman on kidney dialysis who was eating bacon, sausage, eggs, and fatty portions of steak to improve her failing kidneys. She sincerely thought this approach would help her. I did not argue to the contrary. Her dignity was more important at that time. She appeared in such deteriorated health that compassion was the most honorable action. Explaining why this fatty approach would not work would have been futile and degrading to someone whose life had a very short future.

Understanding the reasons why a high fat diet from animal products depletes health rather than promotes better health establishes a foundation of knowledge for making good dietary choices for life.

Not all fat is the same. Fat from animal products creates health issues, cholesterol and heart problems, and diabetes. It in no way can reverse any type of disease. Fat from olives, coconut, wild-caught tuna and salmon, and nuts and seeds, however, do offer many health-boosting components. Your body needs healthy fats for the liver to function properly.

All animal, fish, and poultry consumption is acidic to the body, and this as illustrated on the Potential Renal Acid Load (PRAL) List.

The positive numbers represent the acidic load on the kidneys. The negative numbers are alkaline and do not create an acidic load on renal function.

The more acidic the foods, the greater the risk of stones and disease. The acidic values assigned to the foods were made prior to genetically modified (GMO) agricultural products. For example: the whole milk value on this chart does not represent the more acidic value an updated chart would assign.

US conventional milk contains by-products and additives that create an additional acidic renal load.

The chart remains valid in comparing food items and their positive or negative impact on kidney disease. It can also illustrate that persons developing stones often choose more foods from the acidic portion of the list.

PRAL LIST

ACIDIC FOODS

Meat and Meat Products | Fish

Lean Beef	7.8	Cod Fillet	7.1
Chicken	8.7	Haddock	6.8
Canned, Corned Beef	13.2	Herring	7.0
Frankfurters	6.7	Trout	10.8
Liver Sausage	10.6	Milk, Dairy, Eggs	
Lunch Meat	10.2	Buttermilk	0.5
Lean Pork	7.9	Low Fat Cheddar	26.4
Rump Steak	8.8	Gouda Cheese	18.6
Salami	11.6	Cottage Cheese	8.7
Turkey Meat	9.9	Sour Cream	1.2
Veal Fillet	9.0	Whole Egg	8.2
Sugar and Sweets		Egg white	1.1
Milk Chocolate	2.4	Egg Yolk	23.4
Cake	3.7	Hard Cheese	19.2
Bread, Flour and Noodles		Ice Cream	0.6
Mixed Grain Rye Bread	4.0	Whole Milk	1.1
Rye Bread	4.1	Whole Milk Pasteurized	0.7
Mixed Grain Wheat Bread	3.8	Parmesan Cheese	34.2
Wheat Bread	1.8	Processed Cheese	28.7
White Bread	3.7	Whole Milk Yogurt w/Fruit	1.2
Cornflakes	6.0	Whole Milk Yogurt Plain	1.5
Rye Crackers	3.3	Beverages	
Egg Noodles	6.4	Pale Beer	0.9
Oats	10.7	Coca-Cola	0.4
Brown Rice	12.5	Legumes	
White Rice	1.7	Lentils	3.5
Rye Flour	5.9	Peas	1.2
White Spaghetti	6.5	Fruits, Nuts, and Juices	
Whole Grain Spaghetti	7.3	Peanuts	8.3

PRAL LIST

Sugar and Sweets

Honey	-0.3
Marmalade	-1.5
White Sugar	-0.1

Vegetables

Asparagus	-0.4
Broccoli	-1.2
Carrots	-4.9
Cauliflower	-4.0
Celery	-5.2
Chicory	-2.0
Cucumber	-0.8
Eggplant	-3.4
Leeks	-1.8
Lettuce	-2.5
Mushrooms	-1.4
Onions	-1.5
Peppers	-1.4
Potatoes	-4.0
Radishes	-3.7
Spinach	-14.0
Tomato Juice	-2.8
Tomatoes	-3.1
Zucchini	-2.6

Beverages

Draft Beer	-0.2
Stout Beer	-0.1
White Wine	-1.2
Red Wine	-2.4

ALKALINE FOODS

Legumes

Green Beans	-3.1

Fats and Oils

Margarine	-0.5
Olive Oil	0
Sunflower Oil	0

Fruits, Nuts, and Juices

Apple Juice	-2.2
Apples	-2.2
Apricots	-4.8
Bananas	-5.5
Black Currants	-6.5
Cherries	-3.6
Grape Juice	-1.0
Hazelnuts	-2.8
Kiwi Fruit	-4.1
Lemon Juice	-2.5
Orange Juice	-2.9
Oranges	-2.7
Peaches	-2.4
Pears	-2.9
Raisins	-21.0
Strawberries	-2.2
Watermelon	-1.9

Beverages

Cocoa	-0.4
Coffee	-1.4
Mineral water	-1.8
Tea	-0.3

US conventional milk contains by-products and additives that create an additional acidic renal load.

The chart remains valid in comparing food items and their positive or negative impact on kidney disease. It can also illustrate that persons developing stones often choose more foods from the acidic portion of the list.

Nature produces its own grocery store. In the healthy fats section, wild-caught salmon, tuna, and sardines take center stage. These items are accompanied by olives, coconut, avocados, raw nuts, and seeds.

The body is a complex and amazing healing machine. Providing it with proper hydration and nutrition helps it fight disease and repair damage.

When you buy an avocado, it is exactly that. You can identify what it is and that it came from a tree. When you buy processed meat, for example, it contains a list of unsavory chemicals that render it a danger to your health.

Eating wild-caught salmon, packed with healthy fats and nutrients, is highly regarded for its contribution to better health. Bacon and sausage, on the other hand, are not recommended for consumption when you are in good health.

To reverse potential kidney disease and stones, consuming a diet of 80% alkaline foods and 20% acidic foods provides an acid-base balance. This approach promotes health for every system in the body.

SODA

It is a common misconception that caramel coloring is the ingredient in soda that contributes to kidney stone formation. While it may have some minimal effect over long periods of time, it is not a significant contribution.

Phosphoric acid and high fructose corn syrup are the major ingredients in soda that contribute to kidney stone formation. These unnatural components also impair digestion and cause dehydration. Drinking more soda than water in a day can significantly increase the risk of creating stones.

The average total carbohydrates in a 20-ounce bottle of a cola soda is 65g. To equate total carbohydrates into the amount of blood glucose being metabolized in the bloodstream, follow this calculation:

Total carbohydrates divided by 4 equals teaspoons of sugar

For this example:

65g / 4 = 16.25 teaspoons of sugar

One 20 ounce bottle of soda metabolizes into an extraordinary amount of blood glucose fostering diabetes complications and kidney issues.

This amount of sugar, without any other foods or drinks, creates an emergency for all the systems in the body, not just the pancreas. The organs must shift into overdrive to rid the body of synthetic toxins, produce elevated levels of insulin, and force the kidneys to manage their filtration duties to clean the blood and save a life.

Soda is an inferior carbohydrate that derails all aspects of normal bodily function. It is a manmade, wildly toxic formula that significantly adds to the formation of kidney stones and more than 100 other health issues.

After reading this book, if you have any soda at home and no longer wish to consume it, soda makes a great toilet cleaner, helps break down diesel fuel on clothing, and can remove rust off metal.

Eliminating soda…

Soft drink consumption in the United States dropped for the 13th year in a row! In 2018, Americans consumed nearly 39 gallons per person as compared to 53 gallons in 2000. The US has the highest soda consumption rate in the world.[4]

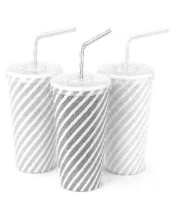

SODIUM

The human body must have sodium to live. It is a tricky subject in food production. The Nutrition Facts Label placed on packaged foods indicates the amount of sodium per serving, but not all sodium is helpful inside the body.

Let's look at the chemical formula for certain sodium components in foods.

Sodium	Na
Sodium nitrate	$NNaO_3$
Sodium nitrite	$NaNO_2$
Sodium chloride	NaCl table salt
Trisodium phosphate	Na_3PO_4

Sodium bicarbonate	$NaHCO_3$
Sodium sulfate	Na_2SO_4
Sodium hydroxide	$NaOH$
Sodium stearate	$C_{18}H_{35}NaO_2$

This chemical formula comparison is simply to visually demonstrate some ingredients in processed foods that are not commonly known and understood. What is all this sodium? Is it good or bad for me?

Each sodium compound (there are many more that are not listed) either helps or hinders the body's proper functioning. Table salt and sea salt are sodium chloride. Humans need between 1800–2000mg daily to keep living and breathing. Any amount over that is excess. The kidneys must work harder to remove it.

Excesses of any type limit proper digestion and kidney function. The toxic material in the bloodstream exits the body through the kidneys, bladder, and urethra.

If these organs are not performing at the highest level, a crystal-like sediment remains, and stones begin to form.

People consume products containing sodium, but it is not all a usable, recognizable substance to the body. Sea salt, pink salt, and other unadulterated forms of sodium help the body perform every function from blinking the eyes to breathing.

You need sodium to survive. High sodium may contribute to stone formation, especially if you are consuming more sodium nitrates and nitrites than sodium chloride. A very low sodium diet can cause restricted functions of all body systems and may result in heart attack or death. Adequate real sodium is essential for human life.

The sodium portion of a high sodium diet does not necessarily cause stones, but the synthetic foodstuffs with corrupted forms of sodium in them do help to create stones.

CITRUS FRUITS

There is a distorted belief that all citrus fruits are acidic and can cause kidney stones. Citrus fruits may appear to be acidic, but they become alkaline inside the digestive system. Kiwi fruit has a potential renal acid load (PRAL) of -4.1. This number means that kiwi fruit has a negative acid load on the kidneys. It has a positive alkaline result of 4.1. Oranges are -2.7 and lemon juice is -2.5. While it may seem odd, the negative numbers have a positive, alkaline impact on kidney function and, therefore, decrease the potential for stones.

The alkaline quality and the beneficial vitamins and minerals in citrus fruits make them *stone inhibitors* rather than contributors to stone creation.

Citric acid in lemon, lime, orange, grapefruit, tangerine, pineapple, strawberry, raspberry, and cranberry, for example, become alkalizing foods that reduce the acidity in urine, promote health and provide essential nutrients for kidney health overall.

With acidosis being the major factor identified in stone creation, consuming fresh fruits and vegetables full of alkaline properties should register at the top of the food choices list if your goal is significantly reducing the risks of kidney stones.

CAFFEINE

Caffeine only contributes to stones when it is excessive or combined with other factors. A cup of black coffee is made from coffee beans grown on a tree. A highly caffeinated, lemon-lime flavored soft drink with chemical additives and high fructose corn syrup is not comparable to a cup of brewed coffee. The two drinks create different and opposing actions in the body.

Consuming freshly brewed coffee while staying hydrated will not contribute to kidney stones. The same is true for loose leaf teas containing caffeine. These naturally caffeinated beans and leaves can offer extraordinary health benefits attributed to their antioxidant properties.

Raw cacao is also a naturally occurring source of caffeine. Cacao is known as a highly nutritious superfood packed with catechins and antioxidants. Because it is raw, it does not contain the sugars and additives found in processed chocolate

In comparison, sodas and energy drinks are synthetic, unnatural commodities placing an unnecessary strain on the kidneys and the rest of the body's systems. It is not the caffeine alone creating the stone issue, it is the substance the caffeine is added into that wreaks havoc on the kidneys.

Energy drinks combined with caffeinated sodas and coffee can create an issue more alarming than kidney stones: Heart attack and even death.

A 2014 Review in the *American Journal of Cardiology* demonstrated the connection between energy drink consumption and cardiovascular issues. The review highlighted that the increasing number of visits to the emergency room are directly related to energy drink consumption. From 2004 to 2007, emergency room visits related to energy drink consumption more than doubled to 20,000 visits annually. Additionally, the review said most of these cardiovascular complications from energy drinks can be attributed to the high amounts of caffeine in these products.[5]

Caffeine **consumed in moderation** is generally considered safe. Continued high dose consumption of caffeine can be dangerous to your kidneys and all other organs. After all, caffeine is categorized as a psychoactive drug.

TAP AND HARD WATER

The idea that tap and hard water causes kidney stones is very interesting. The highest incidence rate of kidney stones remains in the USA, even with the Safe Water Drinking Act standards for removing dangerous contaminants from the drinking water.

Hard water is described by the United States Geological Survey as "high in dissolved minerals, largely calcium and magnesium."[6] Higher levels of calcium and magnesium in hard water have been proven to reduce the risk of heart disease.

In a study conducted in West Bengal, India, dated May 2018, investigating hard water and kidney stone formation, the results concluded that hardness was not a significant factor in stone formation, but the amount of water consumed *was* a key factor. This study reports that dehydration plays a more predominant role in stone creation than the type of water.[7]

One complicated situation when addressing tap water in the US is the inability to filter prescription medication residue from the reuse water supply. While it is assumed that very small amounts of these contaminants will cause no identifiable harm, there is no guarantee this statement is correct.

Many over-the-counter and prescription medications are known to contribute to the formation of kidney stones. Since each town's 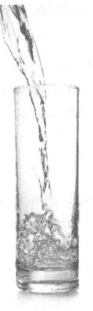 resources are so different from the next, it is difficult to compile a national standard for medication contamination levels in the water or the specific health correlation.

Research published in the *Journal of Environment Science and Technology* from Johns Hopkins University reported the discovery of highly toxic compounds in chlorinated water.

The study analyzed the effects of chlorine mixed with drinking water and revealed previously unknown by-products. In this laboratory test, two BDA compounds were identified, and are known carcinogens.[8]

The Environmental Working Group, a nonprofit organization, released new information addressing a certain class of chemicals in drinking water nicknamed *forever chemicals*. The Per- and Polyfluorinated Substances (PFAS) do not disintegrate. Eventually, they find their way into the water supply and ultimately into our bloodstream.[9]

A piece of information slightly more concerning is the Fact Sheet on PFAS maintained by the Centers for Disease Control and Prevention (CDC). A National Health and Nutrition Examination Survey (NHANES) gathers information about PFAS through collecting blood samples and measuring contaminants in the clear portion of the blood known as serum. The latest findings reveal:

CDC scientists found four PFAS (PFOS, PFOA, PFHxS or perfluorohexane sulfonic acid, and PFNA or perfluorononanoic acid) in the serum of nearly all of the people tested, indicating widespread exposure to these PFAS in the U.S. population.[10]

Tap water is contaminated with more junk than we want to acknowledge as a nation. The tools required to effectively analyze thousands of chemical compounds and the intensive filtration system required to extract all of the damaging content from the water supply does not exist. The cost of upgrading water systems across the country would be exorbitant.

Currently, there are no conclusive studies that show tap water causes kidney stones. The Safe Water Drinking Act lists 91 contaminants that must meet quality standards for drinking water to be considered legally safe for consumption. There are over 60,000 chemicals being used in the US and eventually enter the water supply.[11]

When a chemical is recognized as dangerous on its own, it remains a danger in tap water. While it is of a lesser volume, it will still accumulate inside the bloodstream and require filtration through the kidneys. Humans need water to survive. Find a source that you feel safe drinking and stay hydrated.

CHAPTER 6

KIDNEY STONES IN CHILDREN

As eating habits have shifted away from homemade meals and fresh produce to convenience foods and bottled drinks, the potential for kidney stone issues in children has sharply increased.

According to an article titled, *Pediatric Urolithiasis,*

The study reported that the incidence of kidney stones has increased among young patients (26% increase in 5 years for those 15-19 years of age).[1]

A 26% increase within five years is astonishing! It is a statement of our inability as a country to properly provide the basic education and nutritional requirements for our children.

Knowing that kidney stones are a symptom indicating that more serious health issues are eminent unless dietary changes are made, you can only imagine the severity of childhood disease if the next five years has a 26% increase!

While this astonishing increase illuminates the 15 to 19-year-old age group, children as young as 5 years old are being treated for kidney stones.

It all begins with dietary choices for basic nutrient balance. The same major contributors to kidney stone formation in adults contribute to stones in children: processed junk food.

Antibiotics, steroids, over-the-counter and prescription

medications compromise digestive function and help create dehydration, placing a heavier load on kidney function.

The challenge with children is helping them enjoy healthy foods and consuming water instead of sugary drinks. Kidney stones are the body's announcement that something is not working very well. Both parents and children need to recognize this meaningful message.

Children suffer headaches from dehydration. Often, headaches are the first symptom announcing that increased hydration is necessary. Kidney stones are another symptom. People are led to believe that drinking anything made of water is hydrating. When the body is struggling, plain water is the fastest, easiest way to hydrate.

Water helps flush out toxins without the body having to filter the additional synthetic and artificial ingredients loaded into the soda, juice or other beverage.

Fresh fruits and vegetables provide water content as well as bountiful nutrients. Snacks of watermelon, apples, kiwi, or mangoes deliver hydration, and the vitamins and minerals in these fruits help fortify every cell for better health.

Tips for parents and children:

Drink some water every two hours. It will increase hydration and help reduce the risks of headaches and kidney stones.

Help the body stay hydrated with a fresh, juicy piece of fruit at breakfast, lunch, or snack time.

Balance processed foods with fruits and vegetables. Some of childhood meals such as burgers and fries or chicken nuggets and macaroni and cheese can increase dehydration.

Encourage children to choose a vegetable to eat first. A small portion of steamed broccoli, raw carrots or celery, for instance.

Offer fresh fruit or vegetables as an after school and work snack. This way, both parents and children are practicing healthy habits.

Serve juice or soda in a 4-ounce glass and water in a larger, perhaps 8- or 16-ounce glass. It becomes a visual illustration of which drink is more important.

When going food shopping, allow the child or children to choose one new fruit or vegetable to try that week. Once they make a choice, help them learn some facts about it: where is the produce grown and on what type of plant, the vitamins and minerals it contains, and how their choice helps the body. It will help them understand why they are choosing something new.

Here are some guidelines to encourage children to try something new.

If you love it, you can share it or eat the whole item yourself and then describe to everyone at the table why you love it.

If you do not like it, you can share and do not have to eat it but need to verbalize the reasons why you do not like it.

Describing why they like or dislike something can be associated with texture rather than flavor.

Using pineapple as an example, some younger children may enjoy the flavor, but the texture is a bit too intense. Adding a slice of pineapple to water for flavor or a smoothie may be a better way to encourage them to consume this fruit.

Each week the list of "love it" or "it's okay" grows longer. The "I hate it list" does not exist. It establishes the idea that taste buds cannot grow and change. Instead, that list can be labeled, "not for me right now."

Children like to feel important and involved. As they watch the list grow, they can feel a sense of accomplishment and empowerment to improve their health.

Try juicing an orange the old fashioned way, with a manual citrus juicer. It provides an illustration of how much real juice is in the fruit. Children, especially teens, are amazed when they see the results.

Statement from the Kidney.org website:

Kidney stones are found in children as young as 5 years. In fact, this problem is so common in children that some hospitals conduct 'stone' clinics for pediatric patients. The increase in the United States has been attributed to several factors, mostly related to food choices. The two most important reasons are not drinking enough fluids and eating foods that are high in salt. Kids should eat less salty potato chips and French fries. There are other salty foods: sandwich meats, canned soups, packaged meals, and even some sports drinks. Sodas and other sweetened beverages can also increase the risk of stones if they contain high fructose corn syrup.[2]

Young children usually do not take themselves grocery shopping. Childhood kidney stones are a result of the dietary choices being made for them. Those same choices can result in diabetes, heart disease, and potentially kidney disease.

Your decision and approach to making dietary changes, even when they seem small, can help reduce the odds of kidney stone development.

Decreasing the incidence of childhood kidney stones begins

with water, fresh fruits and vegetables, and education at home. Food choices designed for children in the US market contain ingredients that are banned in other countries.

It has been said that it takes a village to raise a child. Sometimes we forget that our children are eating foodstuffs offered to them by grandparents, neighbors, babysitters, and their schools. This social circle may not be aware of how damaging soda, candies, and colorful snacks can be to a child. Educating the adults in the child's village helps validate parental rules and also helps reduce mental confusion for the child about what is healthy. Something to consider.

A new era of childhood malnutrition has emerged. Toddlers are drinking soda and cappuccinos. First graders are taking multiple medications for health issues that can be easily remedied with wholesome foods. Teens are comparing anti-depressants and anxiety medications as if they were trophies. The current trend of synthesized foods, drinks, medications and lack of vital nutrition education is the crux of childhood maladies. The village has truly let them down. Together, we can change that paradigm, one step at a time, one child at a time.

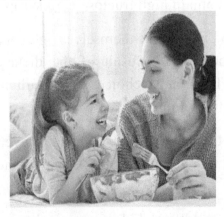

When a child is sick or in pain, it can be one of the most helpless feelings a parent can experience.

As a parent, you have the power to foster the change that can influence your child's healthy life.

CHAPTER 7

ENVIRONMENTAL TOXINS

As if learning that some of your favorite foods and drinks contribute to kidney stones isn't challenging enough, it does not land the same punch as discovering the impact your job or home may have on kidney stones and kidney disease.

One of the major life-saving functions of the kidneys is to filter the blood. Breathing toxic elements or having skin exposed to known contaminants, can register as a kidney stone contributor.

Cigarette smokers experience twice the amount of stones as non-smokers.[1] This fact comes as no surprise, really. Smoking is recognized as a number one carcinogen by the World Health Organization (WHO). It contributes to liver and kidney disease; cardiovascular issues, mouth, throat, and lung cancers; and an extensive list of other health conditions.

Just as inhaling chemicals from smoking cigarettes or vaping disturbs the body's normal systems, breathing pollutants from a variety of natural and manmade substances reacts the same way inside the body.

"Whether you eat it, put it on your skin or inhale it — however something gets into your bloodstream, the liver is going to process it," explains Nancy Reau, MD, a hepatologist (liver specialist) at Rush.[2]

The liver processes it then the kidneys filter it out of the blood.

The incredible human body engages the dangerous toxic exposure we confront every day. Let's break it down.

Your living space.

The numerous chemicals and fumes we choose to believe are safe, compound inside the body as toxic waste. People decided they were safe as individual ingredients, but the kidneys themselves were not consulted. Listed below are commonly used products with chemicals.

- Air fresheners
- Appliance cleanser
- Bathroom cleaner
- Bleach
- Carpet cleaner
- Cooking spray
- Dish detergent
- Deodorant
- Facial cleanser
- Furniture polish
- Hair Care
- Laundry care
- Makeup and makeup remover
- Mold/Mildew remover
- Nail care
- Paint
- Window cleaner

This is a very short list to provide a glimpse into the variety and number of pollutants inside our living area. The best part of this list is that we are in charge of purchasing these items. Less toxic options are available on the market. The next list is less controllable.

When outside, it can be tough to conceive how many toxins are floating into our lungs on any one day. Depending upon where you live can reduce or elevate exposure.

The environmental list includes:

- gas/diesel fumes
- heavy metals
- pesticides
- insecticides
- lawn care applications
- rubber
- cardboard
- plastics
- industrial waste
- cigarette smoke
- e-cigarette vapors
- pet hair and products
- personal care products

These are just a very few items to create awareness concerning the variety of pollutants.

The United States Environmental Protection Agency (EPA) includes 187 pollutants as hazardous.[3] A complete list can be found at epa.gov/haps/initial-list-hazardous-air-pollutants-modifications.

When we consider the sheer amount of buses, planes, helicopters, trains, semi-tractor trailer trucks, automobiles, motorcycles, boats, off-road and recreational vehicles, contributing to air pollution, it evokes a broader vision. Industrial pollution adds another layer. Wildfires, building fires, traffic accidents, floods, hurricanes, tornadoes, chemical spills, adds another layer, and the list goes on and on. Pollution, both air and water, pose an immediate threat to human health and all other living things.

Minimizing exposure within the confines of your living space helps lessen the strain on the entire body. Every function is negatively affected by inhaling pollution particles. Kidneys are the heroes that filter the blood and help sustain life.

Certain occupations are exposed to more intense pollution and hazardous situations than others. Personal protective equipment (PPE) is recognized as a deterrent for exposure, such as masks, gloves, and breathing apparatuses. Both skin exposure and inhalant dangers exist in occupations less likely to utilize protective gear.

Hair and nail salons, furniture manufacturing, new construction projects, sawmills, semi-tractor truck drivers, pesticide applicators, farmers, mechanics, and cleaning services, for example.

To stay healthy in the age of massive pollution, control the areas of your life that you can.

- Eliminate chemical cleansers and consider more natural solutions.
- Get rid of unusable items so the space is easier to keep clean.
- Use a mask when cleaning or exposed to unwanted pollution.
- Stay hydrated and clean up processed food habits.
- Supply the kidneys with the tools necessary to help them keep you healthy.

Eliminating all pollution exposure may not be an attainable goal. Rather, limiting the amount of daily exposure in your immediate environment is a daily process and lifelong challenge.

CHAPTER 8

NATURAL REMEDIES

Wouldn't we all love to own the patent for a quick and easy solution to break up and flush out a kidney stone?

There are some natural approaches to help ease the pain of stones and promote urination, but they have limitations. Certain herbs can interfere or interact with prescription medications. To best address the use of unapproved home remedies for kidney stone issues, let's first review how long it takes to pass a kidney stone and when to seek medical attention.

The starting point for this information begins with the most critical situations first. Here are the **guidelines for seeking immediate medical attention**.

- Inability to urinate
- Temperature 101.5°F or higher
- Sustained, intense pain
- Continued nausea or vomiting
- Bloody or cloudy urine
- Have multiple symptoms
- Have only one kidney
- Are taking medications for advanced disease
- Suffer from kidney disease, diabetes

Any of the above symptoms alone or in combination are alerts that something more serious than just a kidney stone is occurring.

Choose to take good care of you.

For less urgent situations, there are some simple steps to take to help ease the pain associated with kidney stone pressure and to help pass it more quickly.

Small stones, 4mm or less, can usually be passed without medical intervention. For help passing stones faster, try

- Drinking water with freshly squeezed lemon juice
- Taking a teaspoon of organic apple cider vinegar
- Eat a banana, cantaloupe, orange or raisins
- Eat celery, watercress, radish for hydration
- Make a strong tea from dried pipsissewa herb
- Nibble on a fresh parsley leaf
- Using warm or cold compresses can help ease pain.

Now for the reasons why:

Drinking water provides hydration and increases output. Urination is the only way for the stone to exit.

Apple cider vinegar contains acetic acid which helps shrink the stone and thus helps ease the pain.

Lemon juice adds citric acid, which is known to help dissolve the calcium sediment portion of the stone and reduce its size.

Because passing a kidney stone is intensely painful, most people tend to chug water in an effort to pass the stone faster. This effort usually results in losing electrolytes. Eating fruits and vegetables, such as a banana, cantaloupe, orange or some raisins, celery, watercress, or radish, helps stabilize potassium and other electrolyte levels.

Pipsissewa (pronounced Pip-sis-a-wa) is used throughout the

world to help break down kidney stones. A very strong tea is made from dried leaves and consumed throughout the day.

Nibbling on parsley leaf accomplishes several goals. One, it helps increase the volume of urine. Two, it helps raise the urine pH level. Three, it serves as a distraction through the pain and can quell an upset stomach.

Applying a heating pad or cool compress for comfort may help ease the discomfort as the inflamed area of the lower back relaxes a bit from the inflammation. It cannot help the stone pass any faster but can provide a feeling of relief for some time.

Natural remedies can help promote urination quantity while helping to dissolve certain types of stones to the point they can be passed without medical intervention. Stones that are larger than 6mm may take much longer to pass using natural remedies. Medical attention is generally the preferred option due to the severity of pain and the amount of time required for natural remedies to decrease the size of the stone(s).

ESSENTIAL OILS

The list of apple cider vinegar, tea, herbs, fruits, and vegetables on the previous pages have no known negative effects nor do they directly interfere with most medications. However, when introducing essential oils, a list of medication contraindications warrant consideration before use. It is easy to check the essential oil of your choice online for possible warnings, especially if you are taking blood thinners or high dose medications of any kind.

An additional consideration is the possibility of seeking medical intervention for stone removal or pain relief. Please keep in mind that whatever goes onto the skin, or is inhaled or consumed, it is processed by the liver and then the kidneys. The use of essential oil products may potentially complicate or delay medical assistance.

Essential oils, especially food grade or therapeutic quality, offer incredible healing benefits. Some oils can be as strong and effective as medicine. Oregano essential oil is used in commercial chicken farming in lieu of antibiotics, for example.

When dealing with severe kidney stone pain, anything and everything that is known to help reduce the agony and discomfort is implored. Understand your choices and, when in doubt, seek medical attention. Kidney stones that are blocking urine excretion are very dangerous.

While waiting for the stone to pass, it is best to remove certain foods to help reduce the potential of continued contribution to its size. Consider eliminating these items:

- soda and energy drinks
- meat, fast food
- junk food

Kidney stones are painful and complicated. Find a solution that works for you.

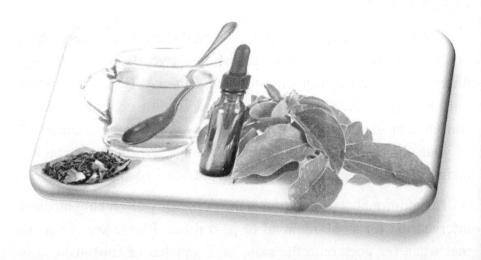

CHAPTER 9

SUMMARY AND GUIDELINES

What to do to reduce your risk of developing kidney stones:

Hydrate with water. Other beverages may offer some level of hydration, but they can also impair kidney function due to synthetic ingredients.

Guideline: Drink more water than other beverages.

Too much animal protein. Fast food "meats" are not really meats in most chain restaurants. They are one-third low-grade meat and two-thirds fillers or are artificially flavored soy protein. Drastically reduce your consumption of these modified animal proteins. They are contaminated, unwanted beyond our national borders, health-destroying substances that create life-altering conditions and disease, including kidney stones.

Guideline: If you must have meat, find a local source of free-range beef or poultry. Eat meat sparingly.

Processed meats are a carcinogen. Bacon, sausage, hot dogs, and salami are listed as a number one carcinogen by the World Health Organization. They are in the same category as cigarettes and plutonium. Deli meats, pepperoni, and kielbasa are not mentioned by name but are classified as processed meats. These products are known to cause colorectal cancer, other health conditions, and contribute to the formation of kidney stones.

Guideline: Eat these products very cautiously, if at all. They are known carcinogens.

High Fructose Corn Syrup is not food. This modified sweetener is added to many processed foods and beverages.

It is cheap and easy to make. It is highly documented for its contribution to diabetes, impaired digestion, compromised intestinal function, and kidney stone formation. Countries around the globe report increased kidney stone prevalence as processed food sales rise.

Guideline: Start reading labels to gain knowledge about products currently being consumed containing high fructose corn syrup. Eliminate as many of those processed items as possible.

Your body makes its own oxalates. Dark leafy greens and tea are not the reason for kidney stones. Yes, there are oxalates in spinach and asparagus, but your body secretes and absorbs its own oxalates as well for proper nutrient assimilation in the intestines.

Please consider this information: most of the persons being instructed to eliminate high oxalate vegetables and real loose leaf tea from their diet rarely consume any of these products. How is it possible that spinach, leafy greens and tea are making stones inside a body that doesn't eat or drink those things? It is not the cause of the problem.

Guideline: You can eat any fruits and vegetables in moderation. Eat a spinach salad on Monday. Red leaf lettuce based salad on Tuesday. Spring mix on Wednesday, etc. Kidney stones are a mixture of habits such as dehydration, lack of vitamin D and calcium, too much animal protein and more. Fresh fruits and vegetables are stone inhibitors and offer nutrients for better health for the whole body.

Consume alcohol correctly. Alcoholic beverages are fermented, and many persons consuming beer, wine, and spirits do not suffer kidney stones because of three habits.

One, they drink in moderation. Two, they drink water while they are drinking alcohol to remain hydrated. Three, they do not mix spirits with juice or soda; rather, it is consumed straight or over ice, thus eliminating the sugar contribution to stones.

Guideline: Alcohol consumed correctly and in moderation does not cause kidney stones. Beer and wine contain nutrients, wine contains high levels of antioxidants and beer, wine and spirits are noted for their ability to lessen the risk of heart disease, stroke, diabetes, and dementia. Again, these benefits are derived when alcohol is consumed in moderation.

Eat some organic raisins. Acidosis is the major cause of kidney stones. Organic raisins are the most alkaline food you can eat. A handful a day is packed with antioxidants, nutrients, and helps reduce acidosis and the risk of kidney stones. If you do not like the taste, add them to water or another beverage to steep.

Guideline: Organic raisins are a safe, delicious food. They promote health and alkalinity to every cell in the body. Eat a few every day. They are a quick, easy way to promote better health.

Frequent urinary tract, bladder or kidney infections.

Both of the components, the bacteria and the antibiotics used to treat the infection, contribute to kidney stones.

Guideline: Take precautions to reduce the risks of infection, stay hydrated, and drink freshly squeezed lemon or orange to help nurture kidney health.

CHAPTER 10

❦

TESTIMONIALS

These testimonials are being shared to help characterize some of the struggles and personal situations people experience relating to kidney stones. Perhaps their journey can help you in a positive way.

From Sammy: Country Boy and Kidney Stones

Look, I'm a country boy. Steak and potatoes, ribs and slaw, pork chops and noodles, chicken and dumplings! The third time I passed a kidney stone, I wasn't sure I was going to survive. Pain? I do mean pain, brother!

I heard about a lady that helped people get to a better place with their health. She told me about uric acid, animal protein, minimizing the amount of meat I ate, and I could not stand to hear another word. To me, vegans were wimps. Like, who doesn't eat meat?

She excused herself, came back to the room, and handed me picture frames with people's stories about changing their food choices and how they got better from really serious disease. After reading one or two of the shorter ones, I just told her the way I was feeling. I could not survive without eating meat.

She asked if I watched football and what team I liked. Heck, I could talk football all day long. I mentioned the Titans, and she said something like, "I cannot believe you ever watched the Titans or know anything about them. A year ago, some of the Titans converted to vegan or mainly vegan." I'm originally from

Tennessee. Saying that about my brothers was blasphemy. I was still on the meat wagon.

"If you want help, I can help you," she said. "If you don't, enjoy your stones." She got up to leave the conversation. I asked if there was another way. She said very calmly, "If you want to stop making stones, you have to address the cause. You have expressed no interest in correcting the issue, so unfortunately, I cannot help you. You must be willing to help yourself." That Dr. Guyer is a tough lady. I realize now that I really did need to hear the truth.

I left. I was dumb, ridiculous, and uninformed. I went home, did some research on the Titans, and felt like a fool. She was right. I was afraid. The only thing I knew, meat, was making me sick. Just like she said stones are just the beginning. Wait until you get the bad news kidney disease.

Long story short, I changed my habits. I eat fruits and vegetables all day long. At night, I eat a small portion of a locally grown organic cow or chicken. NO pork. I loved pork.

Never felt better. Since that day, I've learned a lot about nutrition, water, sugar, disease, how the body works. All thanks to Dr. Guyer for not giving up on me. Didn't pass any more stones, and I'm still cheering for the Titans. Take some advice from a country boy. Back off the meat.

Melissa – Girls Get Kidney Stones

I called in sick and told my boss I was passing a kidney stone. The pain was so unbearable, it was hard to talk. I could tell from the tone of his voice he did not believe me. I was in sooooo much pain. I could not sit or stand or lay down or even take a deep breath.

My next-door neighbor could hear me making sounds of agony

through the walls. She knocked on my door and told me about pipsissewa. She said it helped dissolve stones. I would have done anything to get rid of the pain. I had no insurance. No family in the area. I was scared and exhausted.

She made a tea out of the Pipsissewa herb, squeezed some lemon into it, and I started drinking it around noon. It was awful tasting. I drank it anyway, getting down twelve cups before midnight. I sat in a reclining chair to sleep. I could not lie in bed. I fell asleep, by some miracle, and woke up the next morning with crazy amounts of pressure.

I went to the toilet and passed the stone! It was instant relief! I arrived at work only to be pulled into the supervisor's office for lying about my condition. Women supposedly do not get kidney stones. Luckily, the neighbor that helped me out is a law clerk! I called her on speakerphone in my boss's office, and she railed him to the wall. I went to see Dr. Guyer two weeks later. She explained a new diet plan to help eliminate new stones. I was not very happy about it. I was an athlete on a high protein diet. I played softball.

I agreed to the new diet plan for one month. Holy cow! I did not expect to like the food, but I did. I had more energy and slept better than ever. I recently had a sonogram, and it did not show any stones. I am a very happy camper.

Although a vegan-vegetarian diet does not sound appealing, I am really enjoying the cost savings because meat is so expensive, and I actually love the foods I'm eating. I like the weight loss and my mind is so much more focused. I encourage you to try it. You just might like it. You will definitely like not having any more kidney stones!

From Tony – Let Go of the Meat

Six kidney stones in four years. I was a mess. Grappling for any hope I could find. Then a coworker mentioned changing my diet and seeing Dr. Guyer for some information. I liked what I was eating and who likes to change anyway. Then I got a wake-up call. My employer sent me a final warning letter about my attendance. The next time I was off for illness would be my last working day because I was out of sick time for the year.

Kidney stones run in the family. I can't help that. I felt belittled and betrayed. I had worked there for 18 years.

Turns out, kidney stones don't run in the family, but bad meals do. I was a meat, potatoes, gravy, ice cream, and soda guy. I was ignorant about vegetables and didn't know the names of half of them. But the kidney stone situation was real and getting worse. Like I said, six stones in four years.

Dr. Guyer suggested removing meat and sugar from my diet for thirty days. I think I lost some brain cells when I heard her say that. I was desperate, so I agreed to try it. For the first few days, I hated my life and my condition. I loved meat. I mean, loved meat. I did some research like Dr. Guyer suggested. Guess what? Yep, meat causes kidney stones. I ate salads, baked sweet potatoes, steamed asparagus, wild-caught tuna once a week, fruits, nuts, seeds, sprouts, beans, rice, mushrooms, and olives. By the end of the second week, I started feeling like a new man, but I was too embarrassed to tell anybody. After the month was up, I started convincing myself I could go back to the same habits I enjoyed, Meat, baby, lots of meat! My wife asked me to reconsider. While I was on the diet, I slept better, was calmer, more easy-going, had no indigestion, and we saved about $100 a week in groceries. I lost 23 pounds in 30 days. She did the diet with me and lost 18. Steak, as it turns out, doesn't quite taste the same as it did before we cleaned up.

Today, we are clean, green, carrot-munching machines, full of energy, and looking forward to a brighter future. Two or three months ago, I would not have believed such a change was possible. Let go of the meat. It is not worth it, but you are.

From William: Made of Stone

I'm not good at writing so here goes. Got tired of stones, ER visits, missing work, and pathetic paychecks. Hated feeling scared of not knowing when the next stone would hit. Stopped going to concerts or camping out because I was too afraid of what might happen if a stone hit me.

Met with Dr. Guyer. Hated everything she said. Went home, didn't follow any of the instructions. Then I saw a program on TV about vegan Olympians. There were an estimated 70 vegan athletes at the Winter Olympics. My messed up mind could not conceive of people getting strength eating nothing but vegetables and weeds.

I was wrong with a capital W. Totally WRONG. I decided to try the diet plan for a week. I know this is too much information, but I could go to the bathroom with ease! Big deal to me, not to others. I wrote this testimonial to help someone else that might be in my situation. Sick. Stones. Stuck. Stereotyping vegans. So here is my advice. Take it or leave it.

God made plants. Men made bread. God made fish. Men corrupted animals. God designed perfection. Men filled it with pills. God made me. I need to man up.

Thanks, Dr. G. Without you, I would still be made of stone.

From Brandi and Alan: Hard Lesson to Learn

We owe it to everyone to tell and share this story. I thought kidney stones happened to uneducated, poorly fed people who drank too much or did drugs. My boyfriend and I are college grads living the dream and running marathons. We bought into the high protein, meat, and just a few types of vegetables diet.

Alan got the first stone two days before a big race. I remember being mad about it. I couldn't understand how this could happen. He was cheating on our perfect diet was the reason I came up with.

I got my first stone two weeks later! He was far nicer to me than I was to him. The analysis of the stones was uric acid-based. My sister told me it was because we ate too much meat. Angry and confused, we decided to see the famous Dr. Guyer. We called her the no meat woman.

The way she explained what was happening inside us made sense. After a 45-minute lesson on what and how to eat to eliminate stones and recover health (we thought we were healthy), we left to go grocery shopping.

Still not convinced we should ever eat a carbohydrate; I called a physician friend of mine. She was a runner. When I explained our situation, she just laughed hysterically. She was a vegan.

She said high protein diets are dangerous. Carbs provide energy. Meat weighs you down. She sounded like a repeat of Dr. Guyer's session. Nutrition, hydration, digestion, uric acid, fruits and vegetables.

I hung up and started crying. I researched what I learned about meat. It was clinically substantiated. Too much meat causes kidney stones and a bunch of other health disorders.

We changed our diet. I got the courage to call the people I literally shamed into eating the high protein diet and told them the new information I learned. I didn't want their kidney stones being on my conscience.

For a smart person, I was stupid about food and health. I hope our story in some small way helps save you the agony of kidney stones.

From Gary: This cannot be happening….

For fourteen years, I worked a sixty-hour workweek on salary to climb the ladder of success. I was rewarded with a high paying senior executive position. Happiness was in my corner. We were courting a new corporation for partnership in a large and lucrative project, and I was the man in charge.

On Monday morning, a car arrived to drive me to the airport for the business trip I had anticipated for three months. At the first stoplight, I experienced severe pain. Thinking it was nerves, I continued to the airport. Two miles later, I had excruciating pain so intense I screamed out loud.

The driver insisted I go to the hospital and catch a later flight. I could get some pain medication and relieve my mind. I agreed. We both thought it might be appendicitis.

A scan in the emergency room revealed four kidney stones! The pain was horrible. I had to cancel the trip and was mad as hell. How could I get kidney stones? There was no history of kidney stones in my extended family; I was educated, healthy, ate an appropriate diet and exercised. How could this be possible? I thought drug users got kidney stones.

The doctor said we had to use a procedure called lithotripsy to break up the stones so they would pass. I can only recount that I was in horrible pain and mad at the world. This incident was incomprehensible to me.

My executive assistant told me to contact Dr. Guyer so I could learn some kidney stone information. I smugly told her I would be fine. I was still upset about having stones.

When the executive team got together after my return from the hospital, my elder counterpart suggested I call Dr. Guyer for a consultation. I asked what she could do. I had already passed the stones. They were gone.

He quoted a percentage of patients with recurring stones. I was livid. I do not have kidney issues or health problems.

To get to the point, Dr. Guyer provided information about how to eat and the basic cause of kidney stones. It was different from everything I learned about food. I grew up with the food pyramid. Now she was explaining the pyramid was not correct.

At my follow-up appointment with a kidney specialist, I expressed my concerns about future stones and how to prevent them. He handed me a paper listing the foods I should avoid. They were the same foods Dr. Guyer explained were stone inhibitors. She used the story about astronauts to support her claims.

The foods on the list from the specialist office were not the cause of my kidney stones issues. I never ate those foods. The only valid information I learned through this process was from Dr. Guyer. Eat a lot of fresh organic produce, drink water, limit meat, and be happy ever after.

If you need help, talk with Dr. Guyer. She is a literal library of information on just about every health subject.

My quarter-of-a-million dollar education does not compare to her wealth of knowledge. Eat real foods and be well. Six words of wisdom it took me 48 years to learn and understand.

I hope this story will help you on your better health and no kidney stones journey.

Final Thoughts

Change begins when you have a real desire to accomplish a goal. For most people, their list of accomplishments is already long. Finding a job. Getting married. Renting an apartment or buying a house. Earning a degree. Serving our country. Volunteering. Making a difference in someone's life.

Your good health is priceless and worth every ounce of effort to fight for it. You are the only person alive that can accomplish that goal. You can do this: one healthy bite at a time.

Notes

Chapter 1

1. Glenn M. Preminger, MD, and Gary C Curhan, MD, ScD, "Patient education: Kidney stones in adults," (Beyond the Basics), 2019; uptodate.com/contents/kidney-stones-in-adults-beyond-the-basics>; accessed 15 Jan 2020.

Chapter 3

1. CA Wagner, N Mohebbi, "Urinary pH and stone formation," US Library of Medicine, National Institutes for Health, 2010;

   https://www.ncbi.nlm.nih.gov/pubmed/21170875>;

   accessed15 Jan 2020.

2. BW Turney, PN Appleby, JM Reynard, JG Noble, TJ Key, NE Allen. "Diet and risk of Kidney stones in the Oxford cohort of the European Prospective Investigation into Cancer and Nutrition (EPIC)," US library of Medicine, National Institutes of Health, 2014;

   https://www.ncbi.nlm.nih.gov/pubmed/24752465; accessed 15 Jan 2020.

3. Organic Consumers Association, "Here's why Most of the Meat Americans Eat is Banned in Other Industrialized Countries," 2017; EcoWatch;

   <https://www.ecowatch.com/antibiotics-meat-2454994122.html>; accessed 15 Jan 2020.

4. The Daily Meal (no author specified), "These American Meat Products are Banned Abroad," Huffington Post, 2014; <www.huffpost.com/entry/these-american-meat-produ_b_5153275>; accessed 15 Jan 2020.

5. Roni Caryn Rabin, "Why these food additives are banned in Europe – but not in the United States," 2019; Advisory, January 3, 2019;

   https://www.advisory.com/daily-briefing/2019/01/03/banned-foods:accessed 15 Jan 2020.

6. Sissi Cao. "Americans' Declining Beef Consumption is Worrying Luxury Handbag Makers," Observer, 2018; <www.observer.com/2018/06/americans-declining-beef-consumption-leads-to-less-leather>; accessed 15 Jan 2020.

7. United States Geological Survey, "The Water in You: Water and the Human Body," 2019; https://www.usgs.gov/special-topic/water-science-school/science/water-you-water-and-human-body?qt-science_center_objects=0#qt-science_center_objects ; accessed 15 Jan 2020.

8. Marita Cantwell. "Estimates of Shelf-life of Raw Nuts Held at Different Temperatures," University of California, 2014; <www.ucanr.edu/datastorefiles/234-2753.pdf/>; accessed 15 Jan 2020.

9. Leslie Mann. "Study finds nearly half of Americans not drinking enough water," Chicago Tribune, 2013; https://www.chicagotribune.com/lifestyles/ct-xpm-2013-06-05-ct-x-0605-drinking-water-20130605-story.html; accessed 15 Jan 2020.

10. Chelena Goldman. "This is the Average Number of RX Meds Americans Take Daily," Cheatsheet, 2017;

11. https://www.cheatsheet.com/health-fitness/how-many-rx-

meds-does-the-average-american-take.html/>;

12. accessed 15 Jan 2020.

13. Didia Bismara Cury, Alan C. Moss, Nestor Schor, "Nephrolithiasis in patients with inflammatory bowel disease in the community," US Library of Medicine, National Institutes for Health, 2013;

https://www.ncbi.nlm.nih.gov/pmc/articles/PMC3735273/; accessed 15 Jan 2020.

14. Aviva E. Weinberg, MD, Chirag J. Patel, PhD, Glenn M. Chertow, MD, MPH, and John T. Leppert, MD, MS, "Diabetic Severity and Risk of Kidney Stones Disease," 2013; ncbi.nlm.nih.gov/pmc/articles/PMC3866968; accessed 15 Jan 2020.

15. Yuval Noah Harari, "HomoDeus: A Brief History of Tomorrow," 2017: London, Vintage.

16. Elizabeth Large. "The average American eats 63 dozen doughnuts a year," Baltimore Sun, 2009;

https://www.baltimoresun.com/bs-mtblog-2009-03-the_average_american_eats_63_d-story.html; accessed 15 Jan 2020.

17. Tim Convy. "How many donuts we eat every year," Y98 Radio, 2018; <www.Y98.radio.com/tim-convy/how-many-donuts-we-eat-every-year>; accessed 15 Jan 2020.

18. American Society of Nephrology (ASN), "Reflux and ulcer medications linked to kidney stones and chronic kidney disease," 2016; Science Daily.

https://www.sciencedaily.com/releases/2016/11/16111813035 1.htm; accessed 15 Jan 2020.

19. Kristina Penniston, PhD, "Four Myths about Kidney Stones," 2016; University of Wisconsin-Madison Department of

Urology, https://www.uwhealth.org/news/four-myths-about-kidney-stones/48583; accessed 15 Jan 2020.

20. International Agency for Research on Cancer, World Health Organization Press Release No. 240, October 26, 2015; iarc.fr/en/mediacentre/pr/2015/pdfs/pr240_E.pdf; accessed 15 Jan 2020.

21. Veronique Desaulniers, DC, "New Research Links Excessive Oxalates to Breast Cancer," 2019; Thermography Clinic Ireland; <https://thermographyireland.ie/2019/05/new-research-links-excessive-oxalates-to-breast-cancer/; accessed 15 Jan 2020.

22. Chirag N Dave, MD, "What causes struvite stones in nephrolithiasis?" Medscape, 2020;

https://www.medscape.com/answers/437096-155522/what-causes-struvite-stones-innephrolithiasis; accessed January 15, 2020.

Chapter 4

1. Pietro Manuel Ferraro, Eric N Taylor, Gioranni Gambaro, Gary C Curhan, "Soda and Other Beverages and the Risk of Kidney Stones," 2013; United States Library of Medicine, National Institutes of Health; <www.ncbi.nlm.nih.gov/pmc/articles/PMC3731916/>; accessed 15 *Jan 2020.*

3. Rodney Dangerfield, Successories.com, 2015; <www.successories.com/iquote/author/1506/rodney-dangerfield-quotes/1>; accessed 15 Jan 2020.

Chapter 5

1. National Aeronautics and Space Administration (NASA),

"Using Ultrasound to Zap Kidney Stones and other Health Problems in Space," 2019; <www.nasa.gov/

mission_pages/station/research/news/b4h-3rd/hh-ultrasound-to-zap-kidney-stones> accessed 15 Jan 2020.

2. Calcium Fact Sheet for Consumers, 2019; United States Department of Health & Human Services, National Institutes of Health, Office of Dietary Supplements;

<www.ods.od.nih.gov/factsheets/Calcium-Consumer/> accessed 15 Jan 2020.

3. Friedrich Manz, MD, and Thomas Remer, PhD. "PRAL List," *Journal of the American Dietetic Association*, July 1995, Volume 95, Number 7, 791-797.

4. Emma Bedford, "U.S. per capita consumption of soft drinks 2010-2018," Statista, 2020;

<www.statista.com/statistics/306836/us-per-capita-consumption-of-soft-drinks> accessed 15 Jan, 2020.

5. J., Daniel. "Do Energy Drinks Need Warning Labels?" *Healthy Eating | SF Gate*, https://healthyeating.sfgate.com/energy-drinks-need-warning-labels-12006.html; accessed 15 Jan 2020.

6. United States Geological Survey, "Hardness of Water," < https://www.usgs.gov/special-topic/water-science-school/science/hardness-water?qu-science_center_objects=0&qt-science_center_objects=0#qt-science_center_objects; accessed 15 Jan 2020.

7. Pubali Mitra, Dilip Kumar Pal, Maghusudan Das, "Does quality of drinking water matter in kidney stone disease: A study in West Bengal, India," 2018;

https://www.ncbi.nlm.nih.gov/pubmed/29744472; accessed 15 Jan 2020.

8. Carsten Prasse, Urs von Gunten, David L. Sedlak,

"Chlorination of Phenols Revisited: Unexpected Formation of **α,β-Unsaturated C4-Dicarbonyl Ring Cleavage Products**," Science Daily, 2020;

<www.sciencedaily.com/releases/2020/01/200128142744. htm>; accessed 15 Jan 2020.

9. Sydney Evans, David Andrews, PhD, Tasha Stoiber, PhD, and Olga Naidenko, PhD, "PFAS Contamination of Drinking Water Far More Prevalent Than Previously Reported," Environmental Working Group (EWG), January 22, 2020; <www.ewg.org/research/national-pfas-testing>; accessed 15 Jan 2020.

10. Centers for Disease Control and Prevention (CDC), Per- and Polyfluorinated Substances (PFAS) Factsheet, Last reviewed April 2017;
<www. cdc.gov/biomonitoring/ PFAS_FactSheet.html> accessed 15 Jan 2020.

11. Charles Duhigg, "That Tap Water Is Legal but May Be Unhealthy," New York Times, December 19, 2009; <www.nytimes.com/2009/12/19/us/17water.html> accessed January 15, 2020.

Chapter 6

1. Sahar Fathallah-Shaykh, MD, Richard Neiberger, MD, PhD, Mary L. Windle, Luther Travis, MD, Craig B. Langman, MD, Deogracias Pena, MD, "Pediatric Urolithiasis," 2018; <www.emedicine.medscape.com/article/ 983884-overview>; accessed 15 Jan 2020.

2. National Kidney Foundation, Inc., "Kidney Stones"; https://www.kidney.org/atoz/content/kidneystones; accessed 15 Jan 2020.

Chapter 7

1. Mohammad Reza Tamadon, Mohammad Nessaji, Raheb Ghorbani. "Cigarette Smoking and Nephrolitiasis in Adult Individuals," Nephro-Urology Monthly, 2013 winter; 5(1): 702-705.

2. Gregory Rauch, MD and Nancy Reau, MD. "The Truth about Toxins," Rush University Medical Center Health & Wellness, <www.rush.edu/health-wellness/discover-health/truth-about-toxins>; accessed 15 Jan 2020.

3. United States Environmental Protection Agency. "Initial List of Hazardous Air Pollutants with Modifications:" <www.epa.gov/haps/initial-list-hazardous-air-modifications>; accessed 15 Jan 2020.

Bibliography

American Society of Nephrology. "Reflux and ulcer medications linked to kidney stones and chronic kidney disease," *Science Daily* (November 18, 2016)

Bedford, Emma. "U.S. per capita consumption of soft drinks 2010-2018," *Statista* (2020).

"Calcium Fact Sheet for Consumers," United States Department of Health & Human Services, Office of Dietary Supplements of The National Institutes of Health, (December 6, 2019).

Cantwell, Marita. "Estimates of Shelf-life of Raw Nuts Held at Different Temperatures," *University of California* (2014).

Cao, Sissi. "Americans' Declining Beef Consumption is Worrying Luxury Handbag Makers," *Observer* (June 11, 2018).

Carsten Prasse, Carsten et al. "Chlorination of Phenols Revisited: Unexpected Formation of **α,β-Unsaturated C4-Dicarbonyl Ring Cleavage Products**," *Science Daily* (January 20, 2020).

Convy, Tim. "How many donuts we eat every year," *Y98 Radio*, (May 17, 2018).

Cury, Dídia Bismara et al. "Nephrolithiasis in patients with inflammatory bowel disease in the community," *International Journal of Nephrology and Renovascular Disease* (July 29, 2013).

"Dangerfield Quotes," *Successories*.

Daniel, J. "Do Energy Drinks Need Warning Labels?" *Healthy Eating | SF Gate*

Desaulniers, Veronique, DC. "New Research Links Excessive Oxalates to Breast Cancer," *Thermography Clinic Ireland* (May 26, 2019).

Duhigg, Charles. "That Tap Water Is Legal but May Be Unhealthy," *New York Times* (December 19, 2009).

Evans, Sydney et al. "PFAS Contamination of Drinking Water Far More Prevalent Than Previously Reported," *Environmental Working Group* (January 22, 2020).

Fathallah-Shaykh, Sahar, MD et al. "Pediatric Urolithiasis," *Medscape* (May 5, 2018)

Ferraro, Pietro Manuel et al. "Soda and other beverages and the risk of kidney stones," *Clinical Journal of the American Society of Nephrology* (2013).

Goldman, Chelena. "This is the Average Number of RX Meds Americans Take Daily," *Cheatsheet* (November 30, 2017).

Harari, Yuval Noah, *Homo Deus: A Brief History of Tomorrow*. London: Vintage, 2017.

"Hardness of Water." *United States Geological Survey.*

"Initial List of Hazardous Air Pollutants with Modifications," *United States Environmental Protection Agency.*

International Agency for Research on Cancer, World Health Organization. Press Release No. 240 (October 26, 2015)

"Kidney Stones," National Kidney Foundation, Inc. *Kidney.Org.* (Version undated).

Mann, Leslie. "Study finds nearly half of Americans not drinking enough water," *Chicago Tribune* (June 5, 2013).

Manz, Friedrich, MD, and Remer, Thomas, PhD. "PRAL List." *Journal of the American Dietetic Association (1995).*

Mitra, Pubali et al. "Does quality of drinking water matter in kidney stone disease: A study in West Bengal, India." *Investigative and Clinical Urology* (March 2018).

National Aeronautics and Space Administration. "Using Ultrasound to Zap Kidney Stones and other Health Problems in Space," (2019).

Organic Consumers Association. "Here's Why Most of the Meat Americans Eat Is Banned in Other Industrialized Countries," *EcoWatch* (July 9, 2017).

Penniston, Kristina PhD. "Four Myths about Kidney Stones," *University of Wisconsin-Madison Department of Urology*. (May 19, 2016).

"Per- and Polyfluorinated Substances (PFAS) Factsheet," *Centers for Disease Control and Prevention* (2017).

Preminger, Glenn M, MD, and Curhan, Gary C, MD, ScD. "Patient Education: Kidney Stones in Adults - Beyond the Basics," *UpToDate* (October 10, 2019).

Rabin, Roni Caryn. "Why These Food Additives Are Banned in Europe – But Not in The United States." *Advisory*. (January 3, 2019).

Rauch, Gregory, MD, and Reau, Nancy, MD. "The Truth about Toxins," *Rush University medical Center Health and Wellness.*

Tamadon, Mohammad Reza, et al. "Cigarette Smoking and Nephrolitiasis in Adult Individuals," *Nephro-Urology Monthly* (2013).

"The Water in You: Water and the Human Body," *United States Geological Survey.*

"These American Meat Products Are Banned Abroad." *HuffPost* (April 16, 2014).

Turney, BW, et al. "Diet and risk of kidney stones in the Oxford cohort of the European Prospective Investigation into Cancer and Nutrition (EPIC); *European Journal of Epidemiology* (2014).

Wagner, Carsten A, and Nilufar Mohebbi. "Urinary PH and Stone Formation." *Journal of Nephrology*, (2010).

Weinberg, Aviva E et al. "Diabetic severity and risk of kidney stone disease." *European Urology* (2014).

ABOUT THE AUTHOR

For over 20 years, Dr. DK Guyer has been helping people recognize the potential for reversing disease through a natural, holistic approach to nutrition. Regarded as the nation's leading medicinal tea designer and renowned natural health expert, Dr. Guyer holds a dual doctorate in Natural Health and Nutrition. She founded an organic tea and herb company in 2004 and currently serves as the CEO of Guyer Holistic Education.

Dr. Guyer combines decades of experience with an unparalleled passion for sharing education about what really causes disease and how to change your health for the better. A high energy lecturer, Dr. Guyer's attendees leave laughing and eagerly prepared to embrace a new approach to health.

Residing in South Central Pennsylvania, Dr. Guyer is a business owner, speaker, author and educator.

Made in the USA
Las Vegas, NV
21 September 2023

77917737R00062